THE PERFECT MATCH

by
Steve Pizzolato

The Perfect Match by Steve Pizzolato

Published by Steve Pizzolato
Copyright © 2022 Steve Pizzolato

For permissions, contact: theperfectmatchbook@gmail.com

Cover Design by Ted Wright

ISBN: 978-0-578-36382-0

This book is dedicated to my wife, Nancy Pizzolato, who encouraged me that I was never too old to write a book. She also put up with me ignoring her during the writing of this book and my constant rehashing of what I wrote each day. Special thanks go to early readers and advisors, including my mother, who gave me my love of reading, and my older brother and former 6th-grade teacher, Greg Pizzolato, who still teaches me. Rhonda Moloney, whose life and "theories" ignited my creativity. Plus, I would like to thank the Sunset Country Club Book Club women for offering to read the book and supply critical feedback for improvement and Ally Nikolaus for helping me in the early stages of the book production and publishing.

Finally, and most importantly, I dedicate this to Frank Zuccarelli, who, along with his wife Sue, whose real-life journey of being a transplant recipient inspired the idea. May they live the long and healthy lives they deserve.

DISCLAIMER

While some local St. Louis businesses, hospitals, educational institutions, and locations are real, any activity or involvement with those facilities or people working at those facilities described within this book is purely fictional.

SYNOPSIS

Frank Esposito has an incurable lung disease and needs a double lung transplant in months to survive.

Arch City Transplant Center opened in St. Louis, MO, challenging cultural and ethical paradigms in end-of-life decisions and the organ transplant business. Brilliant doctors run ACTC: Dr. Alex Finnegan and Dr. Ellen James-Calabrese, who will push each other and society to create a company that will be worth billions of dollars, but unbeknownst to Dr. Calabrese, Finnegan is using his colleagues, investors, and the poor as pawns to get what he truly wants.

While Finnegan seems unstoppable and untouchable, a series of carjackings and murders investigated by St. Louis homicide Detective Rhonda Simon threatens Finnegan's plans. With the help of a compassionate organ transplant nurse and one of Finnegan's business partners, Detective Simon realizes her current cases connect to a crime more significant than she initially thought.

Meanwhile, Dr. James-Calabrese's ex-husband, Vinnie Calabrese, will stop at nothing, including jeopardizing his ex-wife's career to get his brother-in-law, Frank, the lifesaving double lung transplant he needs.

The Perfect Match was inspired by first-time author Steve Pizzolato's brother-in-law's battle for a double lung transplant. The book is a crime-filled adventure of murder, everyday people, ethics, the U.S. healthcare system, the 'My Body, My Choice' movement, and how it is all connected to impact our future in more ways than we can imagine. The novel set in St. Louis will introduce readers to a city known nationally for its crime statistics but also one with world-class health institutions, old-world neighborhoods, and parks, making it a great community despite its national reputation.

TABLE OF CONTENT

CHAPTER 1

While brief, the early evening June thunderstorm dropped the temperature and humidity down to a more bearable level for a quick run. It was too early, even for late spring in St. Louis, to experience temperatures of 90 degrees with daytime humidity in the high 70s. Lacing up his running shoes, Kenny Thorton yelled out to his girlfriend Layla that he would be back in about 45 minutes. His usual route took him from the Central West End area of St. Louis, across Kingshighway, and into Forest Park. Except for crossing the six lanes of traffic on Kingshighway, a thoroughfare that separated the peacefulness of the park from the noisy hospital complexes, once he got into the park and its many running trails, he would have no concern with cars. Kenny usually ran a 5-mile loop. This evening, he kept a good pace, feeling refreshed by the lingering droplets of rain from the quickly departing cumulus clouds moving east, away from him and towards downtown St. Louis. He would do five miles at around 10 minutes a mile, but with a cooling breeze and more energy than he had felt in a while, he thought he would push himself this evening and try to complete his course in a little better time. There weren't many runners or bicyclists to congest the paths, and Kenny thought either the isolated thunderstorms or the soon setting sun kept them away, which was fine for him because running was the only time in his day that he felt unburdened with his life's choices.

The park, as beautiful and popular as it was during the day, was not a place to hang out as the darkness of nighttime approached and took hold. Kenny followed the path on the park's outer edges, giving him a more direct route to the stop he had to make. The path gave him the best viewpoint to see approaching runners or nosy people. He ran west paralleling Lindell Avenue, with its stately mansions that were originally state houses for the 1904 World's Fair. The park's golf course, the History Museum, and tennis facilities were on his left. As he passed the halfway point, he came to a slight rise in elevation, which always got his blood pumping a little harder during this part of his run. Once he reached the crest of the Hill, the path would split into a fork, with the right side being the main path, wider and more open with fewer trees, while the left side went into a darkened and heavily treelined area. Most runners avoided the left fork because, while perfectly safe during the day, it did immerse you into a temporary canopy of trees that blocked out the sunlight, giving you a sense of isolation. Also, popular urban myths would have you believe that this path would take you deeper into the woods, supposedly in years past, the haven for the depraved and perverted, secretly engaging in immoral sexual acts or drug deals. Kenny did not believe the folklore and knew he would have a better chance of finding a golfer looking for his lost golf ball from the fairway on the other side of the woods than he would stumble across two men in a compromising position.

About 200 yards after he first entered the darkened area of the path, he turned slightly left into a small, somewhat underused picnic pavilion that he knew would be empty this evening. He soon stopped to catch his breath, untie his shoe to remove a pebble, and innocently greeted another person, the only other visitor in the pavilion area, who, like Kenny, was in runner's clothes. The greeting was brief as the runner, not sweating profusely as Kenny, knelt beside him and quickly slapped into Kenny's palm the smallest of packages, a 2" by 2" clear baggie with white pills. Kenny took the package, slipped it in his shoe, slipped his shoe back on, and continued down the path.

His fellow runner casually walked out of the pavilion in the other direction, wondering why anyone would sweat to get the "runner's high," as they call it when getting high could be reached by taking a simple little pill. Running to stay healthy seemed like a waste of time to him, and guys hooked, like Kenny Thorton, had so little time left.

Leaving the pavilion area, Kenny reached the main path and followed it east back towards his home. As he ran east, the ground rose high enough to see the St. Louis skyline and the Gateway Arch, six miles away. Kenny never got tired of this sight and never got tired of the drugs he just picked up. He also mused at the notion of a runner's high. It was more like a runner's pain, especially at age 48. Every step he took while running was painful due to a bike accident he had ten years back. Kenny could blame, as he always did, the bike accident that got him addicted to opioids. However, he had the means and intelligence to avoid the addiction that so many others less fortunate than him could not shake or avoid altogether. His mental anguish caused by the steep fall his life and career had taken, as well as the physical pain he had due to the injury, would soon subside after he had the chance to empty his shoe and enjoy the contents of the baggie.

CHAPTER 2

St. Louis' citizens are good at murder. The cops, though? Not so good at catching the murderers or getting a conviction if the case makes it to trial. It seemed that after the Michael Brown case in Ferguson in 2014, everyone was afraid of offending the criminals, those who were working hard to make murder, not baseball, our national pastime – not just in St. Louis but in the entire country. With summer approaching, the citizens of St. Louis placed their bets on whether the city would have more murders than St. Louis Cardinal wins.

The 89th homicide in St. Louis in 2021 occurred on June 17th, a few days before Father's Day. What a great Father's Day gift for two men this weekend. Either they lost a child through senseless murder or eventual imprisonment. The Cardinals had only 35 wins this summer and were a bad team, so the easy money was on murders vastly outpacing the Card's win total in 2021. Detective Rhonda Simon was a 30-year police veteran, hardened by a tough personal life. Detective Simon's life began on a hardscrabble piece of land in rural Missouri, and she continued through failed marriages lost partly by the violence she saw in her job, whose demons she could not chase away at night. She believed St. Louis would easily break the 2020 murder number of 263, one of the highest totals in years, fueled by gang drug-related battles. The heat of the St. Louis summer was starting to heat the sidewalks and heat up the arguments, the tempers, the anger. With the heat comes short fuses, and short fuses are usually put out, at least temporarily, by gun violence. Temporarily because, as Detective Simon knew, the gunshot victim she was presently looking down on probably was the shooter in another murder, perhaps a day or two earlier. This murder was revenge for that shooting. Of course, two days from now, retaliation for this shooting will happen. Short fuses and even quicker trigger fingers will rule this summer.

One more death towards the march to over 200 killed, another violent year for St. Louis. Detective Simon was becoming numb to it all, but her job was to investigate and solve as many murders as possible. However, with 30% of the murder cases still open and unsolved, she set her bar for success extremely low.

Looking at the body, Detective Simon sighed with a mixture of hopelessness and just being damn pissed off and tired. She used her forceps to pry a bullet lodged in the bedroom doorframe. Before the bullet eventually ended here, it passed through the chest cavity of one, William Burroughs, a 28-year-old drug dealer. His specialty was opioids, but any drug he could cut, mark up, and sell to his customers was a good drug. If Burroughs were a white-collar entrepreneur, he would be written up in the Harvard Business Review as he knew a lot about product laddering, customer churn, and channel distribution. He liked to move his diverse customer base up from prescription opioids such as OxyContin or Vicodin to more potent choices such as Fentanyl and Heroin. He had no long-term customers because when he first sold to them, they may have been 17, but their time as a customer would only be a handful of years, and then they would be gone, through death or prison.

The drug roller coaster was an intense and scary ride but usually short. While Burroughs had a lot of customer churn, customers were never in short supply for long. Burroughs was not picky about his customer base. A 17-year-old white girl from affluent Chesterfield in West St Louis County had the same color money as a 25–year-old gang banger from the city streets. They both had the same life expectancy, but the gang banger might die from a gun before an overdose, but if they kept using, they would both suffer an early death. Business was always good, and if he had competition, they would not last long, not in his hood. They had two choices when competing with Big Willie, as he was known on the street. Find a new neighborhood, or be carried to the morgue. But a few days before Father's Day, William Burroughs, both fatherless and an absentee father, would no longer be an entrepreneur in drug trafficking. He would not be seeking more customers but instead be joining some of them in the grave, most probably in hell's afterlife.

Detective Simon looked down at William Burroughs, lying in a pool of blood. She had seen many times what damage a bullet causes after it passes through the chest cavity of a 250lb man. Unlike Hollywood's depictions, a bullet from a Smith and Wesson 9MM, traveling at 900 mph, does not travel a straight path through the front and out the back of a body. It explodes, tears blood vessels, bursts bones into fragments, and sears skin. As it leaves the body, the bullet carries muscle, tissue, bones, and a torrent of blood. It enters the body with life and goes almost always with death, usually in about three seconds.

And the blood is not concentrated in a small diameter like on T.V. It splatters across an entire room on the ceiling, walls, drapes, lamps, and doorframe. William Burroughs was no longer a solid mass. He was entrails, and the inside of this home on Adelaide Ave., in the O'Fallon neighborhood of north St. Louis, was serving today as an artistic canvas for murder. Detective Simon observed this most recent canvas, wondered who the artist was, and assumed it was a person known in the neighborhood as 65% of the murders in St. Louis occurred in north St. Louis. The shooter could be a former drug associate looking to get a more significant share of his cut, a former friend who decided he wanted a little taste of Big Willie's supply, or maybe Big Willie's woman.

Or maybe Big Willie was in the wrong place at the wrong time because, in north St. Louis, you were always in the wrong place at the wrong time, sometimes even if you were in your home minding your own business. The news media always described killings like this as random, but Detective Simon knew they were never random. There was always a trail, depending on how hard she wanted to look. Because it was her job and nothing more, Detective Simon was looking for evidence of a crime that probably would never be solved or investigated very thoroughly. Certainly not cared about by the public beyond when the news cameras were on while police interviewed witnesses or grieving family members who cried out in anguish. As always, there were plenty of "potential" witnesses. Thirty minutes before the neighbors called 911 reporting gunshots, a party was going on. Thirty-five minutes after the 911 call, the place was empty, and despite having at least 20 people fleeing the property, there were none to be found when Detective Simon and the St. Louis Major Case squad gathered on the scene.

They would interview witnesses, but these were secondhand witnesses. They were either scared older people hiding behind darkened shades in their homes or the unfortunate young family man or woman whose only crime was to live in this low-cost, high-crime neighborhood. Hopefully, they will achieve the American Dream and get out before they or their children fall victim to another random shooting. For now, they were living in the American Nightmare. When the criminals came out, the good citizens of this neighborhood would hope to see the sunrise before the 2:00 a.m. sirens, and police cruiser lights awakened them unnaturally but never unexpectedly. They served as witnesses but witnesses whose memory and eyesight faded as the interview questions began. While no decent human in the neighborhood wanted these crimes to continue, few cared about today's victims, so while helping the cops may seem noble, keeping quiet seemed safer. Besides, when the next killing occurred in about three days, no one would remember or care about William Burroughs, including the cops. By then, his spot in the city morgue drawer will be replaced by someone else, and his spot on the street corner selling drugs will soon be filled by the next man up.

CHAPTER 3

The summer of 2021 was not any different from years past. St. Louis had a lot of negativities pointed in its direction. Murder. Drugs. Racial unrest. The big three of urban decay. Since everyone must keep score in America, if you were keeping score, St. Louis was supposedly number one on the national lists of most violent and sinful cities, full of vices and temptations. Vinnie Calabrese believed some vices like drinking, gambling, prostitution, and recreational drug use were ok, and if someone did not get hurt, these vices were harmless. If society was becoming woke, Vinnie was certainly still asleep. Murders, while not being an actual vice, were certainly driven in some cases by human emotions of jealousy, envy, and rage, perhaps fueled by sex and drugs. Vinnie never bothered to be concerned about the growing St. Louis murder rate because, statistically or culturally, he rationalized it.

In his mind, the statistics were skewed as they only counted murders in the declining and small population in the city of St. Louis. If they included total murders in the entire metropolitan area, including suburbs, the St. Louis region would not even place in the top 50 U.S. metros. Culturally, Vinnie, like many of his other entitled 64-year-old white male friends, thought, *What the hell, those getting murdered and those committing the murders were predominantly young black men, so in a way, the problem was taking care of itself.* At some point, those doing the killings and those being killed would cancel each other out. Problem solved. He was bothered, however, by the increasingly large numbers of younger kids caught in the crossfire. It seemed to Vinnie that if the black community did not seem to care by keeping their mouths shut when they knew something about the shooter's identity, why should he care? However, despite real or perceived shortcomings and problems in St. Louis, it was a good town, and Vinnie was proud of it.

Vinnie Calabrese prided himself on his Italian heritage and the linkage he felt to his hometown St. Louis. He was a third-generation Sicilian-American. His grandparents entered the country in the early 1900s, not via Ellis Island in New York, where most immigrants entered the country but from the Port of New Orleans. His grandparents, and he assumed other relatives, traveled up the Mississippi River to eventually find what would become their adopted homeland in the New World. Many stayed in New Orleans because the southern climate seemed more like their Sicilian home in Palermo, while others made it to Memphis, St. Louis, and finally Chicago. Vinnie heard the stories about the difficulty his grandparents faced in the early 20th century while they immigrated to a strange new country. They left behind their homeland to come to the United States and settle in unfamiliar and unwelcoming surroundings. As much opportunity America offered to those who assimilated, it ate up and spat out those who did not.

On June 18th, before the summer heat and humidity began to take an unshakable hold of the city streets and inhabitants, Vinnie awoke at his customary 6:30 a.m. Vinnie lived on Edwards Street in the Italian residential district in St. Louis, referred to locally as The Hill. The Hill is a smaller, quieter version of Boston's North End or New York's Little Italy. While the well-known St. Louis Gateway Arch landmark could be seen in the distance several miles east of The Hill, the grittiness of downtown was a world far away from Vinnie's slow-paced and reasonably safe neighborhood. The Hill was home to two famous baseball players, Joe Garagiola and Yogi Berra. It was also home to some second-rate mobsters: the Michaels, Giordano, and Leisure families. All long deceased and forgotten. Vinnie's home was a shotgun style, long and narrow and so straight a bullet could pass through the front window and exit the rear without hitting a wall. It was made of a heat-holding red brick, as many homes were in this neighborhood. Back in the day, St. Louis was one of the largest brick-producing cities in America. The Italians that settled in The Hill worked tirelessly in the brick factories for their pursuit of the American Dream.

St. Louis was a lot of good things, Vinnie still believed. Despite its hardships and undeserved national reputation, Vinnie loved St. Louis, partly because of the collection of neighborhoods, like The Hill, each with its own identity and personality. The Hill was a group of modest brick homes passed down from generation to generation, with a few knockdowns for those who wanted to build a larger home on two lots. Fortunately, the knockdown craze which swept over other St. Louis neighborhoods had been kept relatively in check, as most of the neighbors were vehemently opposed to any change to the neighborhood character. Anyone who got permission to build a larger new home probably was a long-standing Hill resident or Hill restaurant owner and got a pass from the residents because of that status.

As he did most days, Vinnie started his day by walking to the Missouri Baking Company to grab a Cornetto, an Italian breakfast pastry, then onto Shaw's Coffee for an espresso. There was no Starbucks within miles of The Hill, which made Vinnie smile every morning. After picking up a copy of the St. Louis Post-Dispatch newspaper, another aging symbol of St. Louis' greatness, Vinnie settled on a chair outside Shaw's. Like all local papers in the country, the Post-Dispatch had become a shell of its former self. Started by Joseph Pulitzer, the family behind the journalism Pulitzer Prize, the Post currently consists primarily of ads and about 36 pages of content. Vinnie was only interested in reading two sections this morning, the Sports and the Metro section, which mainly focused on crime and death.

He instantly turned to stories about his beloved St. Louis Cardinals baseball team. This summer, they were playing like crap once again. Their cheap-ass billion-dollar owners, the Dewitts, refused to sign a big splash, big bopper, free agent. Or as Vinnie suspected, the free agents refused to sign with us. St. Louis was not a glamorous town and could not compete with more cosmopolitan cities, also wooing these baseball superstars. After checking the box score of last night's game, lamenting the lack of clutch hitting, or any hitting for that matter, Vinnie glanced at the remaining sports section, confirming the Cubs, the Cardinal's primary rival lost the night before. Vinnie quickly flipped the paper to the metro section, focusing on the crime beat. The Cardinals' coverage and crime beat seemed to be equal in coverage. Of course, the Cardinals only played 162 games during a season, but the crime season was 365 days a year. Today, there was the usual assortment of stories: protest over the presence of a statue from 150 years ago, the nightly carjacking featuring a 14-year-old with a gun about half his size, drag racing crackdowns on Washington Avenue in the downtown corridor, and the previous day's murder victims.

By Tom O'Halloran: St. Louis Post Dispatch, June 17th, 2021:

The St. Louis Major Case Squad investigated the shooting death of William Burroughs, age 28, of North St. Louis. Burroughs was believed to have been murdered by unknown assailants at approximately 9:00 p.m. at 267 Adelaide, in the O'Fallon neighborhood of North St. Louis. The homeowner could not be identified, but shortly before the killing, a large gathering of nearly 20 people took place at the home.

Detective Rhonda Simon of the Major Case Squad is investigating the incident, and according to Detective Simon, no credible witness has stepped forward to identify the assailant. Burroughs was a 28-year-old black man, 6 feet 4 inches in height and approximately 250 lbs. According to Detective Simon, the victim was killed by a 9MM Smith and Wesson at close range. The Major Case Squad is asking witnesses to call their anonymous tip hotline at 1-866-371-8477 (TIPS) to report any possible suspects of the crime.

"Well, one more down and out," Vinnie said a little too loud, interrupting the anonymity of the morning coffee crowd at Shaw's. He thought to himself; this *is such bullshit. No one is going to call that hotline because nobody values life anymore.*

CHAPTER 4

Dr. Alex Finnegan was a freak of nature. Physically, at 6' 4", he possessed the combination of a pro quarterback's physique with movie star looks that a woman may call smoldering. Finnegan's thick black hair accompanied dark blue eyes and a stubbled beard on his square jaw. His physical prowess took a back seat to his intelligence. He finished top of his medical school class at Washington University in St. Louis. After residency and working for a few years, he went into the MBA program at Northwestern University's Kellogg School of Business, combining two esteemed degrees from first-class universities. At 48, Dr. Alex Finnegan could accomplish anything, and his never-satisfied thirst for power, money, and fame, would take him anywhere he wanted to go.

After a successful career as a surgeon and in business as a venture capitalist, Dr. Alex Finnegan started Arch City Transplant Center, a privately owned transplant business. Alex wanted to start ACTC for two reasons. One, he wanted to change how society looked at the two critical components of a transplant: how someone chooses to die and to allow the donor to decide who gets their organs. The second reason: he could make obscene amounts of money in the process. The money came with power, and perhaps more than any of his other goals, gaining power was an aphrodisiac Alex could not ignore.

Today, however, after a long day of dealing with investors in the Transplant Center, the only thing he wanted to do was to go for a run through

Forest Park. As one of the largest urban parks in the United States, commonly referred to as the *Heart of St. Louis*, its 1300 acres, about twice the area of Central Park in New York City, and its eastern border began just a few hundred yards west the hospital complexes and Arch City offices on Kingshighway.

Alex knew the park well and took off heading west, past the Steinberg ice skating rink, around Jefferson Lake, and then ran parallel to the park's 9-hole Highland Golf Course on Clayton Road. He then turned right to run past the Jewel Box, featured in Tennessee William's play, *The Glass Menagerie,* then around the Muny, one of the oldest outdoor theater venues in the United States. His run finally ended at the top of Art Hill, which led to the St. Louis Art Museum and one of the best views in the city. Catching his breath, though he wasn't winded, Alex took in the eastern view over the Boathouse Lagoon and its paddle boats. Beyond the outer reaches of the park's eastern boundary sat the fashionable Central West End neighborhood, and further east, finally to an unobstructed view of the Gateway Arch.

This view reminded Alex of the many large city parks in the capitals of Europe. He never got tired of this vantage point. His gaze, however, pulled back from the horizon and narrowed as he focused on a beautiful young woman clad in black yoga pants and a tank top. She ran along the paths around the Grand Basin and toward him on Art Hill, her blonde hair pulled into a ponytail.

To Alex, women, like business, medicine or life, were to be pursued with a vengeance, probably why he never married as he knew he would never be faithful.

While Alex never had a shortage of women to date, his favorite pastime was meeting them while running through the park. He wanted his physical attributes to be the initial attraction before the women labeled him a wealthy and successful doctor and entrepreneur.

Alex took off racing down Art Hill, trying to catch up with the woman, but he may have met his match in stamina. She proceeded at such a quick pace that Alex found himself languishing further and further behind. So far back, he decided perhaps this was a challenge to meet her on another day.

CHAPTER 5

Unlike Alex Finnegan, Frank Esposito was not a physical freak of nature. He was more of a loving life kind of freak. Frank had unbridled optimism regardless of life's challenges. He had an unrestrained joy in life that he shared with friends, family, and neighbors. In a cynical world, Frank was unique in his pureness. No one would confuse him with a former pro quarterback. Frank was everyman. Navigating raising a family and managing a career had its ups and downs, but he savored each day regardless of its complexity.

Frank was at a stage in his life where he began to value his free time with his wife Sue, their three adult sons, and now their grandchildren. He appreciated family time more than worrying about finishing the next project at work. While needing a few more years to work and a few more dollars to save, Frank was a long way from retiring, and he was realistic about his priorities. At 5'7" in height and slightly overweight, primarily due to the savory Italian dishes and desserts Sue whipped up, he could use some exercise. He got in a three-mile walk almost daily around his neighborhood in Highland, Illinois, a small town about 50 miles east of St. Louis. Beyond the occasional small glass of homemade Italian wine on special events and holidays, Frank tried to live a very healthy life. So, it was a slight surprise to him that after one of his daily walks, he felt much more winded than usual, attributing it to high humidity on a summer evening and perhaps some dust stirred up from the nearby cornfields. He had just turned 60 and had yet to schedule his annual physical, but nothing he felt that night caused him to accelerate making the appointment with his doctor.

CHAPTER 6

Detective Simon used her mandatory 24 hours chasing down leads, typically dead ends, on the murder of William "Big Willie" Burroughs. She reported her progress to Lieutenant Tarallo, her immediate supervisor on the Major Case Squad.

"Ring up number 89, Lieutenant," she yelled out from her desk in the bullpen area of the St. Louis Police Headquarters in the heart of downtown. With no response, she continued talking. "Any bets on where and when number 90 occurs?"

The betting on murder victims was a little stress avoidance game she and the other detectives in Police District 4 occasionally engaged in as they tracked the yearly death toll. This year it was quickly on pace to be over 200 murders.

There was no need to bet on the victim's race or the weapon of choice. The SLMPD homicide report showed that 90% of the murder victims in the city of St. Louis were unfortunately black, and the weapon of choice was almost always a gun. Also, there were no bets placed on the suspect as nearly 30% of the cases in the city remained unsolved after a year. Simon was sure the bleeding-heart liberals would crucify her and her other detectives for making such a mockery of the loss of life. She knew they would think differently than her if they spent a couple of nights on patrol with her or paid a visit to a postmortem victim. But liberal outrage, indifference, and fading interest would occur two days after a crime was committed. Most people would go on with their lives, not caring about the victim, the families, or the ever-growing burden laid on the cops trying to solve unsolvable crimes. "Simon, I got another one for you," Lieutenant Tarallo yelled out after stirring from his office for a cup of hours-old coffee. *I guess number 90 is ready to be investigated,* Simon thought.

"Lieutenant, before I go out, did I win any money on 89?" Without hearing an answer, she grabbed her keys and headed out the door to check out the latest canvas of death and determine who the artist was this time.

Traveling quickly, Detective Simon raced along Olive Blvd. westward towards St. Louis University and its beautiful urban campus just a few miles west of downtown. As she listened to the radio directing her towards the scene, all she could think of was, *please don't let this be some poor coed raped and murdered.* Especially a coed from out of town, a story sure to be picked up by local and national media, further adding to the pounding St. Louis takes on its crime rate. As much as the crime and citizen indifference weighed on Detective Simon, she was a local gal and still had a lot of pride in her city.

As she pulled up to the corner of the Budget Car rental location just north of Olive, east of Garrison, she could smell the BBQ cooking at Pappy's, a wildly popular BBQ place with lines of locals and out-of-towners cueing up by 10:30 a.m. Pulling into a side alley next to the Budget lot, Detective Simon walked up to a motley congregation of people, unfortunately, made up of fellow cops, reporters, and EMTs, all the usual workers at a crime scene. They were all huddled around a 2010 silver Ford Explorer. As she pushed her way through some beefier co-workers, likely regular Pappy's customers, she glanced at the victim, not a coed, thank God, and probably not a student at the university. She was looking at a scrawny, in life and now in death, 30-something meth head with a few teeth missing and, by the looks and smell of him, a few missing weeks of showering and laundering. *Homeless?* Rhonda thought at first, *but why was he in a car?* He had what looked like a shiny new needle protruding from his veiny left arm, and his dead eyes looked up at Detective Simon with satisfaction that he got one last rush.

A probable heroin overdose was not that unusual for the demographics in this neighborhood. Still, there was a large amount of dark red blood, by this time congealing, left over from a wound around the victim's abdomen. Detective Simon pulled back his flannel shirt, the clothing of fashionable homeless drug users on a 95-degree summer day. To her surprise, she found a bloody gaping hole in his abdomen, where his kidney was once occupying. She had never in her 30 years on the streets seen anything like this. Was this man killed for his kidney? Was this some sort of gang payback ritual of which she was unaware? She would let the coroner decide on the cause of death, and while an overdose would not make the news or headlines, a kidney cut out of a body would. Covering the victim with a sheet, she thought *no one would win the death pool on the city's 90th murder.*

CHAPTER 7

Vinnie, now retired, woke up every morning wondering what day it was. Most of his friends who had been retired for years had told him that you genuinely are retired when you cannot remember or care if it was a Tuesday or Saturday. It was a Tuesday, but Vinnie realized it did not matter as he spent his days doing the same routine. Wake up too early to shake away his nightly hangover, grab a coffee and pastry, catch up on the local news, and maybe return a few texts or emails to guys in his golf group to set up a match for the day or weekend. Vinnie's day was a mixture of boredom and mischief, usually influenced by how much booze he drank and how deep he went into depression over his divorce. However, Vinnie woke up today with a surprising and anticipated variation: he had lunch plans with his ex-wife Ellen.

Getting lunch together was not that unusual for Ellen and Vinnie. Thanks to Ellen's generosity in the divorce, she paid for her and Vinnie's memberships, albeit now separately, at Sunset Country Club, a 100-year-old private club perched high on the foothills overlooking the start of the ancient Ozarks Mountains, 30 miles west of downtown St. Louis. They were bound to run into each other from time to time at the restaurant or on the course. Since his divorce, Vinnie used Sunset socially to maintain his golf game and his immediate circle of friends. In retirement, Vinnie found he was more isolated than Ellen, who kept up a busy schedule as a surgeon on staff at Barnes-Jewish-Christian Hospital, known locally as just Barnes or BJC.

For Ellen, Sunset was a professional outlet to stay in touch with the movers and shakers of the St. Louis medical and business communities. During their marriage, Vinnie pushed Ellen to take up golf so they would have some shared interests later in their marriage. Once Vinnie retired, though, he started to shift into second or perhaps third gear, while Ellen's ongoing thirst and drive in her professional career was a root cause of their marriage ending.

Ellen would get exasperated with Vinnie, who seemed to be perfectly content idling and drinking during the day. Ellen could not stand pat for a minute and had not slowed down as she aged. She added more responsibilities to her life and daily schedule.

Vinnie got to the club first. He spent a few minutes bullshitting with his buddies in the Men's Card Room before heading to the restaurant. He selected a table on the outside patio, overlooking the tee box on the first hole and the panoramic view facing west. The table was their favorite. If the conversation slowed, the view let them get lost in it. Looking out at the tee box, Vinnie would place a real or imaginary dollar bet with Ellen on whether the player's initial drive would find the fairway. Whereas Ellen would always comment on the view, wondering how far in the distance her eyes could see and remembering happier times years ago, like 4th of July nights full of fireworks illuminating the sky and the hills on the horizon west of the club.

After ordering his drink, a John Daly, known as lemonade and iced tea mixture spiked with Vodka, Vinnie waited for Ellen's arrival. She was usually behind his arrival by 10-15 minutes due to a long drive and more issues to deal with during her morning. Like clockwork, Ellen strolled onto the patio at 12:15 sharp for noon lunchtime and hurriedly hung up her cell phone as talking on the phone was prohibited in the dining area. Vinnie preordered Ellen her go-to drink: iced tea with lemon and pink sweetener. He could have also ordered her favorite lunch, Salmon Caesar salad, but Vinnie did not need to rush. He had nothing to do that afternoon and would likely hit the driving range or get out on the course for a few holes after lunch. If Ellen were in a hurry, as she usually was, she would order immediately upon seeing Jeff or Scott, the lunchtime waiters. Greeting Ellen as she approached the table was always awkward, even after 34 years of marriage followed by two years of divorce. Vinnie had several options here. One, let Ellen take a seat and, after a few pleasantries, start focusing on the menu, or two, rise to greet her with a hug and direct her to the chair of her choice, which was the one Vinnie was currently occupying. For whatever reason, perhaps the gentle temperature and breeze, the ordinarily hot June day seemed resort-like. Vinnie rose, hugged Ellen, and as if prepared and practiced often, he offered her the chair out of direct sunlight.

Despite the different lifestyles, the slow drift apart, and the eventual divorce, Vinnie and Ellen still enjoyed each other's company. Ellen was dressed very casually for a workday which surprised Vinnie a bit, but even more surprising than that: she called Scott over and ordered a glass of Prosecco, her favorite Italian sparkling wine. Immediately upon greeting each other, they fell into the playful banter that had been the hallmark of their relationship for nearly 34 years.

"Celebrating something?" Vinnie asked.

"No, not celebrating, more like exhaling from a crazy day," Ellen replied. "Do you care to join me, or will I be drinking alone during lunch?"

Holding up his glass, signaling to Ellen that he had already started drinking, which did not surprise Ellen, they waited for Scott to bring Ellen's drink. When they both had drinks in hand, Vinnie asked, "So what kind of crazy day are we talking about, Ellen?"

"Crazy good," Ellen replied. "So good after lunch, let's play nine holes, and I will tell you all about it. I am starved. So, let's eat." Looking up at Scott, "I am in the mood for a burger."

Ok, who has taken over Ellen's body? Vinnie thought. *Drinking at lunch, playing golf with me, and ordering a burger?* Something was up, and Vinnie could not wait to learn about what was going on with Ellen.

CHAPTER 8

A natural, fresh-faced, blonde beauty in her teens, Brooke MacIntosh was even more so as a confident, intelligent, and beautiful adult. She grew up in Kirkwood, a quaint St. Louis suburb as if depicted in a Norman Rockwell painting. It had wide streets, large trees, many turn-of-the-century historic homes, and an old-fashioned but lively downtown main street with thriving restaurants, farmer's markets, and shops.

Brooke graduated top of her class at Visitation Academy, an all-girls, private Catholic high school. Founded in 1833, Visitation was the oldest private girl's school west of the Mississippi River, a notoriety that many St. Louis institutions claimed since St. Louis was one of the oldest cities west of the Mississippi. Since age 10, Brooke helped with her family's restaurant, MacIntosh's. So, instead of going away to college, Brooke attended St. Louis University or SLU as locals called it, just a few miles down interstate 64 east of her home and Visitation. While at SLU, Brooke spent her time focused on completing her nursing degree as quickly as possible. She was driven to accomplish more in the time frame usually allowed, and she also needed money. Every college kid needs money and is in a hurry to live in the real world and make a living, but Brooke needed money because she knew her parents barely made ends meet at their restaurant. Brooke wanted to help them as much as possible, as they had given everything to her and her siblings. After graduating from SLU, she took a job at St. Louis University Hospital and worked nights in the emergency room. There she came face to face with the death and carnage of St. Louis' citizens battered by the drug and murder crisis. Brooke knew the paramedics by name as they delivered patients nightly, what seemed like a war theater's worth of injured or dying to her emergency room entrance. After several years of working at the university hospital, Brooke began to focus her nursing skills on a more significant role in health care as she wanted to run a team at a large trauma center. She entered the Master of Science in Nursing program at SLU and graduated with an MSN degree at age 28. Earning her master's degree, Brooke left St. Louis University Hospital to work at Barnes, the teaching hospital affiliate of Washington University and the largest hospital in Missouri. While Barnes was a national leader in many areas of medicine, Brooke settled in the intensive care unit night shift. Several years later moved onto a pulmonary floor, where she eventually became a transplant coordinator. At age 30, Brooke finally felt all her challenging work and educational commitment had begun to pay off financially and professionally as she could see her life, as she had planned it, begin to take shape.

Brooke was excited to attend a conference on transplants. She had been promoted to become one of the hospital's transplant coordinators. Attending a conference by the American Transplant Foundation was a nice perk allowing her to understand better how the national and local transplants' efforts were coordinated. She had hoped she could have attended the conference held a few months back in Miami, but due to lingering Covid-19 restrictions, she was attending a smaller local conference in St. Louis near the hospital.

The Covid-19 pandemic weighed on Brooke's mind, both professionally and personally. Professionally, her patients were some of the sickest and most vulnerable to any disease. Since many of her patients were awaiting new lungs or had just received their new lungs, respiratory diseases such as Covid could accelerate death. Usually, the ability of the patient to receive a new lung is based on a variety of factors, including overall health, medical history, age, blood type, height, weight, and even a person's lifetime stage. Now Brooke and her team had to factor in Covid-19 as vaccine status became an issue. How likely would a patient who received a new lung survive if they eventually caught Covid? As cruel as it sounded, the ability to obtain a lung or organ transplant that could save your life was, in many cases, weighed against how you lived before needing the transplant.

The impact of Covid on transplants was a break-out session Brooke had highlighted to attend, but Covid-19 was on Brooke's mind as well. The past weekend had been highly stressful for Brooke's family because she and her siblings had a family meeting with their parents about their restaurant, MacIntosh's. The restaurant had not been a gold mine for the family but a steady stream of income for nearly 30 years that paid not for the finer things in life but the important things. They enjoyed a comfortable family home, good education for her and her two sisters, an occasional European vacation every ten years, and frequent trips to Florida or California. But this weekend, the mood was glum as the restaurant had not recovered fully after all the Covid shutdowns. With the kids' help, her parents had weathered multiple shutdowns by cutting costs, including some staff. The entire family pitched in, working unpaid and squeezing enough money from take-out and catering to pay the bills. Fortunately, her parents had always lived modestly and had a small nest egg put away for retirement, which they planned to do after selling the restaurant. But with the restaurant's financial footing shaky, they were unsure if they could find a buyer or if they had enough money to weather this latest unexpected downturn. Their future was murky, and while Brooke's was bright, her concern was on her parents. A family meeting was held to determine how much longer they could hang on and how much of their retirement savings they would want to be used to survive this time.

Brooke and her sisters were adamant they needed to do everything possible to keep the restaurant from closing. "Mom. Dad." Brooke implored them, "You have done everything for us for over 30 years, so let us help you now." Her parents, Steve and Cheryl, disagreed. "Brooke, no. You girls have your lives to live, and our problems should not become your problems," Steve countered. "Besides," Cheryl added, "if the restaurant closes, that will give us more time to take care of our yet-to-be-born grandchildren whenever they come." *Oh, even on the edge of bankruptcy, they played the grandchild card,* Brooke thought, rolling her eyes toward her married sisters Amanda and Jillian. They returned the knowing subtle eye roll.

"We are all working. We have good jobs and can contribute our time and money for the next two to three months, but you are not closing down MacIntosh's. Besides, Mom, if the restaurant closes, where will Jillian, Amanda, and I take your grandkids on Saturday morning to learn about making cinnamon rolls?" Brooke said, smiling, knowing she had used the grandchild card just as smartly as her mother. While this playful back and forth talk did alleviate pessimism in the air, the truth was it would be difficult, if not impossible, to keep the restaurant afloat without help from those sitting around the kitchen table, maybe some luck, and perhaps some divine intervention.

Brooke absentmindedly thought about the weekend's conversation with her parents as she walked into the lecture hall on Washington University's campus, bordering Forest Park's west side. She was scheduled to attend seminars on the transplant industry organized by the American Transplant Foundation in conjunction with several regional transplant centers and hospitals. Usually, a medical conference like this would be at a glitzy locale or hotel. It would run over several days, where speakers and attendees could network, gossip, or view the latest medical transplant technology. But in the era of Covid, Brooke would be attending only with her local medical professionals while most of the speakers were presenting virtually. Sessions like this were being held around the country, with the speakers simultaneously linked into multiple conference halls. During this conference, medical professionals would join in from all the major Midwest cities, including Nashville, Minneapolis, Chicago, Detroit, and Indianapolis.

It was not just a coincidence that these cities were all part of this conference as the transplant business, and it was a business, was becoming regionalized. Patients and donors usually competed among regional transplant centers as to whom would get the donor's organs and which patient would receive the organs. Organizations such as UNOS, the United Network for Organ Sharing have improved the matching rate of donors and recipients so much that despite being in a pandemic, the United States has the best performing donor and transplant system in the world.

While most transplants were done in major medical centers, many patients were in small towns with less sophisticated hospitals.

In many cases, they would lose out on the organ as it may not get to them fast enough to be used, or their local medical team did not have the resources to get to the donor quickly to harvest the organ, or they could not do the operation. For the patient in a rural area to receive the organ, they eventually would need to be airlifted to a more significant medical center. In most cases, the decision was made to supply the organ to a patient already at the medical center if all other factors were equal.

Time and distance were crucial in deciding who would live or die based on their ability to get an organ, which is why rural and urban regions needed to work together to make organ distribution as fair as possible. When a person died or was near death, and they had agreed to donate their organs, they were identified in the UNOS national database and matched against recipients in need. A transplant team would be notified. If the donor were remote from the recipient patient, the team would often fly to the donor by helicopter or private plane, waiting for the donor to succumb eventually. Then they and other teams would take the organs they needed. As morbid as it sounds, there may be several teams, one taking the eyes, others the kidneys, or perhaps lungs and heart. Any organ that can be harvested will be. Then each team would fly back to their respective hospital, and the receiving patients would be taken in for surgery.

The total time window between the donor patient dying until the transplant is performed may be anywhere from 4-8 hours depending upon the organ, some of which only have viability for 2-3 hours. Of course, the patient receiving the organ must be prepared for surgery and have stable vitals to ensure they can still receive it. If not, the entire process, if wasted, is called a dry run, as finding another recipient may be impossible because the best match may be hours away from the harvested organ. While the transplant of organs has been remarkably successful, almost twenty people per day die waiting for an organ match. A successful transplant requires a willing donor, an able host, a skilled medical team, and a lot of luck and timing. A thunderstorm front, delaying flights, may waste a successfully harvested organ.

As a nurse working in a hospital, Brooke always experienced life, when a patient recovers, or a baby is born; or death, when no medical treatment in the world can save a stage 4 cancer patient or a blunt trauma incurred from an auto accident or gunshot wound. As a transplant coordinator, Brooke saw life and death, sometimes with two different patients and their families and, unfortunately, sometimes with the same patient. It was hard to describe the feeling she got working in this role. It was exciting yet sobering. It was joyous yet sad; it was exhilarating yet painful. Brooke loved it.

Brooke perused the list of topics and speakers on her agenda:

10:15-11:15: A donor's family and recipient story: The Winter Family and Jamie Breck

11:30-12:30: The Rural Dilemma: Making the playing field even for rural patients: Dr. Brandy Alderson, University of Missouri Medical Center, Columbia, Missouri

12:30- 1:30: Working Lunch: The impact of Covid-19: Dr. Ezra Sharif

1:30-2:30: Government Regulations and future legislation: Undersecretary of Health and Human Services, Mary Scott, and Congressman Bill Cochran

2:35-3:45: The Perfect Match: Dr. Alex Finnegan, CEO of Arch City Transplant Center

3:45: Program concludes

Brooke had hoped to make all the seminars, but she wanted to sit in on the one by Dr. Finnegan since he would be doing his in person. He was a bit of a local St. Louis medical community legend, personally and professionally. She knew his seminar would be the most provocative as he was known as a maverick in the industry. She quickly scanned her messages, turned off her phone, and went into the first session.

CHAPTER 9

Dr. Jennings spent a minute looking over Frank Esposito's test results before re-entering the exam room.

"How am I doing, Doc?" Frank asked and answered himself. "Yeah, I know. Lose some weight, cut down on the red meat, give up sugar."

"Well, there's always that," Dr. Jennings commented as he peered above the chart, partly reading it and looking at Frank.

"Not going to happen, Doc." Frank went on, "You know how great of a cook my wife is, and besides, food is one of life's great joys."

Dr. Jennings did know how good of a cook Frank's wife, Sue, was. She always had Frank bring Dr. Jennings a tray of freshly made Italian pastries. Dr. Jennings would always thank Frank while admonishing him for the sweets but secretly eating a few as soon as time allowed.

"Well, Frank, your weight is 205, and I think a target is 170 for your size. So, the walking you are doing is a good start. Your BMI is 33, and I want that down to 30, and your blood pressure and cholesterol are a little high but not too worrisome. However, I did notice some issues with the clearness of your lungs. You said you have been more winded than usual after your walks, correct?"

"Yeah, a little bit. But you know I am trying to break that 18-minute walking mile record," Frank said, laughing.

"Well, to make sure you can break the record safely, let's err on the side of caution and have you visit a pulmonary specialist. I will give you the name of Dr. Spiros, a specialist in this field. Let's get you in to see her sooner than later."

With that, Dr. Jennings bid Frank Esposito goodbye, leaving the exam room to let Frank finish dressing. As soon as he did, Frank called his wife Sue. "Good news and bad news. The good news is I can keep enjoying all your cooking; the bad news is I need to see a lung doctor for some reason." Frank left Dr. Jennings' office, not necessarily worried as he was not a smoker and did not work with any toxic chemicals, but as soon as he got to his car, Frank dialed Dr. Spiros' office and made an appointment for the following week.

CHAPTER 10

Ellen and Vinnie finished lunch and then made their way down to the first tee to play nine holes and have what Vinnie hoped would be an interesting conversation, as their lunch left him vexed as to why the sudden change with Ellen. Wine at lunch, taking the afternoon off to play golf, and with him, of all people. It was not as if they did not get along. They did get along well enough for a divorced couple, but Ellen ran in different circles than Vinnie. She wanted other things in her life, driving herself daily to do more, a trait she wished Vinnie had. While she knew he earned his retirement, she also knew he left more on the table. Vinnie would not deny Ellen's opinion of him. Although he had been moderately successful in life and could retire early, Vinnie knew he had more to give, but he did not know how even wondering if he wanted to do more. Vinnie figured any void in his life would be filled by a good meal, a good glass of wine, a good golf score, and maybe, doing something good for someone.

Vinnie playing from the men's blue tees, hit first, and because of his drink, he was loose and hit one straight down the narrow fairway of this opening par 5. Vinnie always knew that when golfing, you had to find the perfect balance between loose and drunk. He started most rounds loose but usually finished them drunk.

Ellen began from the forward tees. Vinnie admired her smooth, effortless swing and how she still looked in her tailored and tight golf outfit. Neither Ellen nor Vinnie dated much after their divorce. However, Vinnie knew that Ellen was still very sought after as he would occasionally catch the leering eye of another club member anytime Ellen walked by while out at the club with her friends. Vinnie always had two emotions when it came to Ellen. A little bit of lust when catching a glimpse of Ellen, like now on the first tee, and a lot of jealousy knowing that other men would love to date her. Vinnie could be a hot head, and he was not sure how he would react to Ellen dating again.

Working their way down the first hole, intermixing a few good shots with bad, they made their way through the next couple of holes just chit-chatting about their round. By the time they got to the fourth hole, a challenging par 3, downhill, over a lake, but in the quiet and isolated part of the course, Vinnie knew he had only a few more holes and maybe an hour or so to get Ellen talking about what brought the sudden change for the day. Ellen, of course, hit a nice easy 6-iron onto the green, and Vinnie put his 9-iron in his usual spot to the left of the green on a hilly landing area. As they finished their hole, Ellen with an easy par and Vinnie with a hard bogey, Vinnie had the opportunity to ask Ellen what was going on.

"So, what was so crazy good about your day that you blew off work, had a drink for lunch, and decided to play golf with me?" Vinnie asked, emphasizing the focus on him, her playing partner.

Ellen laughed, understanding the inflection and bewilderment in Vinnie's question about her golf partner. "Well, it is not that odd that we play golf now, is it?" After all, you taught me to play and love the game."

"Ok, so you want some tips from me. I get it." Vinnie said, knowing that if she practiced more, she would probably be consistently better than Vinnie. "But seriously, what's up? Did someone that you hate die?"

"Funny you used those words, Vinnie. My news has somewhat to do with death and life. But no, no one I hated just died, and that is such a mean thing to say," she said, swatting Vinnie's hand playfully. "You know I don't hate anyone. The truth is that I just got offered an exciting opportunity to work full-time with Arch City Transplant Center. I will be their Chief Medical Officer overseeing the transplant teams."

Vinnie was not listening to Ellen, already thinking about his upcoming tee shot, as his attention span was short and his focus only on himself. Besides, he had no idea what that job entailed, but he assumed it did allow Ellen to combine her medical practice with her love of business.

"So," Vinnie said after hitting his shot 180 yards down the fairway, "how are you going to manage this and your regular job. You know, cutting open people and having their guts spilled out beneath you?" Vinnie had always admired Ellen's skill and success as a surgeon, but the thought of what she did made him nauseated as he hated medicine, sick people, hospitals, and blood.

"Well, I always planned to cut back my medical practice and turn over some of the work to my junior partners. So, this is a good opportunity to do that and start to learn the business side of medicine. I also think Arch City Transplants will revolutionize how we do transplants in this country. They are also giving me share options," Ellen continued after hitting her tee shot straight down the fairway as always.

"Arch City Transplants. Arch City Transplants. Where have I heard that name?" Vinnie asked Ellen as they drove to their golf balls in the fairway.

Before Ellen could answer, Vinnie remembered, "Alex fucking Finnegan. Isn't he the CEO of that company?"

"Yes," Ellen answered, and as she did, Vinnie shanked his straightforward 140-yard approach shot into the woods off to the right. "Damn," Vinnie cursed, as much for his poor shot as for hearing the name Alex Finnegan.

"But that guy is such an asshole," Vinnie huffed as he marched toward the woods to find his ball. "Why on earth would you work with him?"

Ellen did not answer until they were both on the green, Ellen again looking at an easy par and Vinnie faced with a sure double bogey.

"Well, just because you have issues with him at the club doesn't change the fact that he is a brilliant surgeon and businessman. He also is on the cusp of doing breakthrough work in the field of transplants," Ellen added casually as she easily two-putted for her par. "Besides, he is also handsome, which is an added benefit."

That comment caused Vinnie's first putt to go seven feet past the hole, and his next one, two feet short of the hole. Ellen laughed, knowing she had achieved the desired effect to mess with Vinnie's mind and game, although she could care less about Alex Finnegan's looks.

They jumped in the cart and headed towards the next tee box. Vinnie was steaming, unsure whether it was because of the double-bogey six he turned into a triple-bogey seven or Ellen would be working with Alex Finnegan. He decided it was about time to have another drink and go from loose to drunk on the course. Not great for his golf game but great for his mood.

Alex fucking Finnegan, he thought to himself. How the hell could this guy be good at everything? God, he hated that guy. He was the unofficial king of the club, or at least he and his suppliants felt so, as he always won the club championship with his effortless game and single-digit handicap. In business, Alex was very successful. He was also handsome and always had a beautiful woman joining him for dinner. Vinnie thought everything came so easy to Alex Finnegan.

Maybe that is what bugged Vinnie the most about Finnegan. Vinnie had been successful enough, perhaps not as many others in the club, but he always had a blue-collar mentality toward his white-collar success. Vinnie did not come from family money and always worked honestly and hard. Vinnie knew he had a bit of a chip on his shoulder as it was his way of maintaining a competitive edge in business and his personal life. With his 5'7" frame, a bit of a belly, and a thinning hairline, Vinnie was not the best golfer nor as strong of a physical specimen as Alex Finnegan.

Of course, Vinnie was also quite a bit older than Finnegan, so the comparisons were ridiculous, but Vinnie did not like the guy. As Vinnie got older, he conjured up real and perceived grudges against people.

As Vinnie stewed about Alex Finnegan and his deteriorating last few holes with Ellen, he tried to put their conversation in the past. He even congratulated Ellen, showing her a bit of enthusiasm for her new opportunity. As they finished, Ellen, holding out an olive branch, said, "Vinnie, that was fun, and I am sorry I ruined your game with my news and mention of Alex."

"Well, I am not letting that be the reason you beat me again," Vinnie said, totaling up the score. "Let's see, you shot a 46, and I had a 49. It looks like I need another drink and another nine holes. I see Rich and Greg teeing off. I think I will join them, but it was fun playing with you."

"Enjoy the rest of your day," Ellen called out as she walked back towards the lady's locker room, with Vinnie staring at her once again with a bit of lust, jealousy, and now anger as he thought about Ellen working with Alex Finnegan.

CHAPTER 11

Brooke was fascinated by the transplant seminar and the speakers she had heard during each session. Each speaker gave her a unique perspective on transplants that impacted her emotionally and clinically.

The first seminar, featuring a transplant recipient and a transplant donor family, was especially gut-wrenching as it contrasted the initial horror of losing a loved one with the joy of saving lives because of the transplant. There was anger from the donor's family that someone should live while their son died and guilt by the recipient that she lived while someone else died. Over time, the two families agreed to acknowledge each other's presence through letters, emails, and social media contacts. Eventually, they met, and the tears they shared at their first meeting equaled those in the audience hearing their story, including Brooke's.

The second seminar dealt with the inequality of those needing a transplant living in rural areas of the state compared to those who lived near a major medical center, like St. Louis. In many cases, the only way patients had to give themselves an equal chance was to move away from home to a large city to access better medical care and the donor's organs. Moving was a difficult choice for many families because any transplant is not guaranteed, and in the final stages of their lives, would they choose to live away from loved ones? Many decided not to and unnecessarily died based on where they lived. Many moved to a metro area and never received the transplant for other reasons, dying alone, away from home. And some chose to do whatever it took to better their chances of receiving the transplant. Brooke had experience dealing with all these outcomes. During the second seminar, tears again swelled up in Brooke's eyes, recalling some of her patients who died waiting for a transplant that never came.

At this rate, Brooke thought she would be a wreck by the time she completed the last seminars. Fortunately for her, though, the fourth seminar of the day was much drier, both in subject matter and in tears, as it reviewed current and future governmental regulatory issues affecting the transplant industry. While moving forward due to shared real-time databases and improvements in medicine, many people were still dying while waiting for a transplant because of a lack of donors and legislative barriers.

It was an industry that, in Brooke's mind, was bogged down with government complications, red tape, and political agendas or moral guidelines. At least she did not cry during this session but did find herself nodding off a few times as the material, while important, was delivered by two very boring government speakers. During a break between the government seminar and her last seminar, she stopped to get a cup of coffee to wake her up. It was late in the afternoon. Brooke had been up late the night before dealing with last-minute complications of a transplant patient. He was to receive the lungs of a patient that had unfortunately died early in the day and whose organs were being parsed out. Brooke's patient, a young woman, was at the top of the list to receive the donor's lungs, but at the last minute, her vitals weakened, and she was no longer the best candidate to receive the transplant. Not choosing her was a significant life and death decision that, unfortunately, was decided upon in minutes. Her team and the transplant surgeon all huddled, discussing and sometimes arguing the merits of each path. All the time, the patient and her family anxiously awaited the verdict back in their hospital room.

The verdict, driven primarily by the transplant surgeon, who, while having an ego of invincibility, still wanted the best chances for a positive outcome, chose to pass this lung on to the next recipient.

He left, leaving Brooke to share this information with her patient.

Short of having a patient waiting for a transplant die, telling a patient they had been passed up as an organ recipient was the worst part of her job. This decision took a toll on Brooke, which carried on throughout a sleepless night and into these emotionally charged seminars.

The last seminar was of most interest to Brooke as it not only connected the themes of the earlier sessions, but it was being given by a local surgeon, hospital legend, and now CEO of Arch City Transplants, Dr. Alex Finnegan. He was a legend at Barnes. Everyone was in awe of his academic achievements, his surgical skills, his success rate as a transplant surgeon, and now his vision: combining his background in medicine and business to form Arch City Transplants, one of the most transformative private transplant centers happening anywhere in the country, if not in the world. He also had movie-star looks, features not lost on Brooke and most of the females, and probably a few of the male audience members. Brooke had never met Dr. Finnegan. He had phased out of his daily surgical work at Barnes and focused his energy on Arch City before Brooke ever had a chance to meet him. Brooke occasionally caught a glimpse of him going in or out of the hospital but never had the opportunity, or frankly, the nerve to approach him. She took a seat halfway back in the room. She was mesmerized by his insights into the transplant industry's issues and his plan's vision and audacity, which would possibly solve every problem she had heard about in today's seminars. Like most surgeons and CEOs, he displayed an ego that he alone could accomplish this transformation while only minimally referring to the team. He was not short on confidence or cockiness, but she already knew this based on his reputation at the hospital. Dr. Finnegan explained The Arch City Transplant Center would be unique in three areas. The first is they would serve as a whole-body transplant center. He explained that traditionally, when a donor died, transplant specialists would swoop down where the donor was located and take the needed organ, then distribute them to the waiting recipients, who sometimes were hours away. In this scenario and in many cases, time and location were the primary arbitrators of success. Dr. Finnegan rudely described this as the "buzzard on the telephone line" scenario, waiting their turn for a piece of their corpse.

In Dr. Finnegan's vision, if the donor was terminal, death was days or weeks away, or the patient was on life support and would pass in a few days, Arch City would transport them to The Center. Once there, patients would be prepared as best as possible for their future end-of-life donation and the process of matching them with as many donors as they had organs.

In his vision, the donor and the recipient were never more than a few minutes or a room away from each other. As Dr. Finnegan explained, this eliminated time and location as a factor and, like the case Brooke was involved with the night before, would limit the panic of finding a new recipient if things did not perfectly line up. While not referring to this as a donor/recipient assembly line, that was the visual Brooke had, listening to Dr. Finnegan. While Brooke was impressed by this first part of Dr. Finnegan's vision, she and the rest of the audience would be stunned by the second piece of his vision for the Arch City Transplant Center. Dr. Finnegan believed the criteria for matching donor and recipient, historically based on medical acceptance of the donor organ, was missing a significant piece of humanity that he thought would improve the success rate of organ transplants. Finnegan believed that an organ would survive better in the new host or patient if the organ donor and transplant recipient met and knew each other as people before the donor passed. He believed the organ, once transplanted, carried the grieving or anguish of the dying donor, and once transplanted, that anguish would affect the success of its survival in a new host. He further believed the organ recipient, while elated with a chance to survive, always carried guilt that someone died so they would live. His vision was rather than the "buzzard on the telephone wire" scenario; Arch City would become a transitional community where those dying and those needing to live would share that experience with their families. He did not use the words "donor dating site," but that is what image came to mind. Brooke silently chuckled to herself and heard a few bits of laughter in the audience. Lastly, Dr. Finnegan explained the final piece of his vision for The Center, which he knew would leave the audience gasping, booing, or cheering. The ultimate showman, Finnegan, put up one last slide for the audience:

- My Body, My Rights
- My Organs, My Rights
- My Life, My Death, My Rights

He said that the first two changes The Center was undertaking would increase transplants' success rate and the number of usable organs. However, to make a transformational change in the volume of organ donors, it was time that organ donations should come out of the shadows of anonymity. Because he believed donors should be able to choose who their organs could go to, why should they not be able to decide when and how they want to die to facilitate the donation of their organs better? He outlined how the state and national governments, the church, the politicians, and the scientists all have debated the morality of physician-assisted suicide but were not thinking about it in the context of how valuable a person's death could be if they were donating organs. Finnegan argued that if we have complete control of our life, without government interference, the ability to control our death and life-giving organs after death is the ultimate "my body, my choice" decision. Finnegan knew this slide would create chaos in the audience, as it had done so many times in other presentations, with some booing loudly and some standing to applaud. Finnegan said over the noise, "I assure you, my favorite author was not Mary Shelley. And while I loved the Frankenstein movies as a kid and can recite lines of Young Frankenstein, my beliefs are not based on Bavarian folklore or Hollywood. They are based on compassion and the holistic view that the most important people involved in the transplant process are the donor and recipient, and they should have more choices. Thank you for your time."

Brooke sat there, trying to absorb what she had just heard as Finnegan left the stage. She quickly snapped out of her temporary stupor and rushed from the room, hoping to meet him, but by the time she got to the lobby, she saw him walking briskly out the doors, followed by a large group of seminar attendees and others shouting questions at him. "Well, that was certainly exciting," she said only to herself.

CHAPTER 12

Dr. Spiros looked over Frank Esposito's chest x-rays. "Have you ever smoked?" she asked.

"No," Frank replied.

"Have you ever worked with toxic chemicals?"

"Nope."

"Have you ever worked in a coal mine or any area with dust, asbestos, anything like that?" she continued.

"No. I've been an office worker most of my life. Mostly sit in front of a computer," Frank replied.

"Hmm," she said, followed by a silence too long for comfort from Frank's perspective.

She took off her glasses as if trying to ascertain whether to go with the simple layman's explanation or the complex medical explanation. Looking directly at Frank, she said, "Frank, you have Idiopathic Pulmonary Fibrosis, IPF, which is a type of interstitial lung disease or ILD."

"Extraterrestrial lung disease...like ET," Frank said half heartily to lighten the mood and take the tension away from his hands that were unconsciously clenched on the side of the chair he was sitting.

"No Interstitial. ILD causes scarring and inflammation of the lungs. It is a general term for many lung diseases, and you have a specific type called IPF. Frank, it's just medical words and an acronym for lung disease with unknown origins, which is what Idiopathic means. It has caused scarring or fibrosis of your lungs. Pulmonary is another word for lungs," she added.

Silence enveloped the room. No words were coming from Frank or Dr. Spiros.

"So, like pneumonia or a respiratory virus? Something I take antibiotics for?" Frank asked tentatively, knowing he would not get the answer he hoped for.

"No, unfortunately, it is more severe than a virus or pneumonia. IPF is progressive. It is unpredictable, and it is irreversible."

"But can it be treated?" Frank asked. "Irreversible sounds like a death sentence."

"Not necessarily, the disease, as I said, is unpredictable, and the damage to your lungs can occur slower or faster, but since the disease progresses and never retreats, you will be a candidate for a double lung transplant."

"A lung transplant? How can this be happening to me?. I don't even smoke. What do I do next? How long do I have before I need one?" Frank frantically and rapidly asked Dr. Spiros.

While it was hard to tell a patient to calm down after giving them unwelcome and completely unexpected news, Dr. Spiros tried to walk Frank down from the cliff that seemed to be peering over and toward a path of treatment plans instead.

"Well, first, Frank, we know your lungs are compromised. So, we will put you on medicine and oxygen to help you breathe more easily. But this is a long-haul disease, and since we know it is not curable without a lung transplant, the best thing you can do for yourself is get healthier in the eventuality you get a transplant. Frank, as odd as this sounds, the key is to get you physically in the best shape of your life while your lungs fail you. If you do, your chances of being a match for a lung transplant can go way up. You need to get your body in shape for the fight of its life to be eligible for the lungs, and you also need to make sure you are healthy enough to handle the operation and ensure the lungs have the best chance of surviving in your body."

"Ok," was the only word Frank could weakly muster.

Frank left Dr. Spiros' office and looked at his phone for the first time in what seemed to be hours. Several texts from his sons and Sue all asked how the Doctor's visit went. He would talk to them in person once home rather than text. The only person he wanted to talk to now was God, and he did so on the ride home.

CHAPTER 13

Waking up Tuesday morning, Vinnie started the day like he did every day. A walk down the street to grab a pastry, a coffee, then the morning paper. Like most people, Vinnie read most of his news on his phone, but he still liked to grab the paper, more to keep hold of the past before it went away forever.

He thought briefly about his lunch and golf outing with Ellen a few days ago and wondered if that part of his past was gone forever. He certainly enjoyed the day with her, but it had been two years since the divorce, and he had long given up hope that they would somehow reunite, as neither of them had even crossed that emotional threshold. He was sure she did not want to get back together because, in his mind, she had outgrown whatever Vinnie could offer.

Instead of golfing because his back was aching, Vinnie decided to go fishing down at Jefferson Lake in Forest Park. Fishing was the only pastime that allowed Vinnie to take his mind off whatever was troubling him. Two things were worrying Vinnie today. One was his relationship with Ellen. Was it finally over? Was any hope solely in Vinnie's mind, or was she giving him some signal? His second troubling thought was a shocking conversation he had last night with his brother-in-law, Frank, who had told Vinnie that he had been diagnosed with a lung disease that would require a double lung transplant. Vinnie was trying to understand how this could hit Frank out of nowhere. The guy lived the life of a saint, especially when compared to Vinnie's lifestyle. He would visit Frank soon to see firsthand what was happening with him.

As he packed his fly rod in his truck and headed down to Jefferson Lake, he thought a little bit about Ellen and a lot about Frank. Fishing would clear his mind of both problems, and he looked forward to a few hours of quiet solitude. As he stood on the bank of Jefferson Lake, the early morning quietness of the park, contrasting with the bustle of the city just waking up, he noticed the many bikers and runners using the paths that paralleled the lake. As one cyclist sped by, Vinnie heard the roar of a car engine racing up the street, soon followed by the sound of screeching tires. In a large urban park setting, any car going just marginally too fast would only cause someone to notice briefly. So, while he turned back to his fly line in the water, seeing a fish had pulled his strike indicator under the water, he thought about the screeching tires and decided to investigate.

CHAPTER 14

The body count in St. Louis was piling up. So far in 2021, the murder rate was tracking about 30% higher than it had in 2020, and with no end in sight, the heat of the summer began its prolonged assault on St. Louis, its citizens, and its criminals. Desperation is always a secondary cause of murder. In many cases, desperation from losing a lover, desperation to find your next drug score, or desperation to just get some money to survive another day, but in 2021, desperation was more palpable than any of these. That palpability came from citizens having lived through 15 months of Covid. While the restrictions had ended, the disease's impact still lingered in the poorer parts of the city, especially as another surge came through because of low vaccination rates and variants swamping the hospitals. As the summer went along, desperation against the overall battles of life, exasperated by the long-term devastation of Covid on the economy, the family structure, churches, and community, made it seem at times as if oxygen itself was being sucked out of the air the St. Louisans breathed. Putting one foot forward seemed monumental to those losing everything, including loved ones, to Covid.

Detective Simon, who knew the city's violent streets and the people inhabiting them as well as anybody, had sensed the subtle shifting of dread that began in 2020 and continued in 2021. People who had been beaten down in life, pre-Covid, were just now in an accelerated blender of pain and misery. Some of which were their choosing. Simple arguments, usually diffused by a friend or family member, result in a killing. Broken or unrequited love, usually soothed over by some kind words or a supportive night of drinking with friends, was replaced with violence to the former lover. Bickering between husbands and wives, or siblings, usually resolved by cooling off in another room, or a walk in the park, now raged on for days before eventually exploding in violence.

Churches were open, but the sanctuary they offered was limited. Sports venues and teams once were a sought-after and needed distraction from life. They were still not nearly at the capacity and energy they had in the past. Meeting places like coffee shops and restaurants were uncomfortable, too, even if they were fully open. Detective Simon had seen ominous signs of what the summer would bring, and looking at the body at her feet now, and she was hoping this was not another sign of human depravity and numbness towards our fellow humans.

Laying still on the ground and barely breathing was a young man, approximately 20-30 years of age, white, and athletic. His bicycle laid on its side a few yards away, now mangled. Black skid marks around him from car tires were still warm to the touch. The biker was a hit and run victim, as his body suffered blunt trauma because of the collision between his bike and a vehicle of unknown origin.

Although his athletic biking clothes left little room to hold any identification, Detective Simon searched for some in the small pouch strapped underneath the bike seat. She found his phone, license, and a $20.00 bill. His driver's license listed him as Brian Coffman, age 25, living in Clayton, Missouri, a suburb about ten minutes west of the Forest Park bike paths where now he struggled for life. Simon instinctively looked around, as in some cases, the suspect was lurking close by to see their handiwork, but not usually in hit and runs. Had Mr. Coffman been starting or finishing his bike ride? There was no way of knowing as any increase in body temperature could be because of the heat or his exertion after a long ride. Detective Simon knew his body temperature would drop if the paramedics were unsuccessful in staving off death. As the paramedics began feverishly working on Mr. Coffman, Detective Simon moved aside and walked up the street to talk to a surprise guest in her line of work: a witness to the possible crime.

Most crimes in the city never had reliable witnesses. However, this crime was committed early morning when the park started humming with bicyclists, joggers, workers, fishermen, and golfers. Detective Simon approached the witness, surrounded by a combination of St. Louis Police patrol officers and Forest Park Rangers.

Based on the obvious, the witness, a fisherman, had a fly rod in his hand and was wearing a fishing vest. "So, how were they biting this morning?" Detective Simon asked, trying to put the man at ease, who was anything but at ease, as his eyes jumped from the victim, then back to the Detective, and then just blankly at some point in the distance.

"What, what, did you ask?" he answered. But before Detective Simon could respond, he mumbled, "Good, I guess," seemingly still confused as to why he was asked the question in the first place.

Well, so much about putting him at ease, thought Detective Simon.

"So," she said, "let's start with a name."

Silence.

"Your name, sir? What is it?" Detective Simon asked again. She began to think this guy was drunk, but it was only 8:30 in the morning.

"Oh, my name. It's Vincent Calabrese," he finally replied out of his stupor. "But call me Vinnie."

"Italian?" Detective Simon asked, knowing St Louis had a large Italian population, and although a big city, it was just a town of ethnic neighborhoods.

Silence again from Vinnie.

"So, Mr. Calabrese," Detective Simon forged ahead. "Could you tell me what you saw or heard regarding this incident?" She pointed to the cyclist, who was placed into an ambulance.

Then, as if a jolt of clarity or alertness came over Vinnie, he started in on his description of the events at a rapid and random pace.

"I was standing on the banks of Jefferson Lake and saw this guy riding his bike on the path paralleling the lake and Faulkner Avenue. While I usually concentrate on the water, the fishing was slow, so I glanced around, enjoying a nice morning and the scenery and people watching."

Vinnie continued, "I always marvel at how busy the park is and how it allows people of all social classes to enjoy it. You know the park is the best thing about St. Louis, in my opinion. It is so egalitarian."

"Egalitarian?" Detective Simon interrupted, "What does that mean?"

"It means a place where all people are equal. Rich, poor black, white, young, old, liberal, conservative. At a park, we are all equals, and we all equally can enjoy it." Vinnie went on as if now teaching a social studies class instead of supplying a witness testimony on a crime.

"Hmm," Detective Simon said. Mr. Calabrese was neither drunk nor senile, as she initially suspected, but perhaps a more profound thinker and potentially a better witness than she thought he would be when she first started this conversation.

"Go on, sir, but take your time and slow down," Detective Simon said, giving him more respect.

"Well, as I said, fishing was kind of slow, and I normally keep a watchful eye out myself because when I am down here early, you never know if you're going to cross paths with someone wanting to cause trouble. Although the park is a safe place, people are unpredictable."

Detective Simon nodded in agreement.

"The guy on the bike rode by and headed north towards the Steinberg Skating rink, towards the park's wildflower areas, ponds, and streams. It is the most beautiful part of the park but also one of the more isolated parts." Detective Simon nodded in agreement as she knew the park well.

Vinnie continued, "Well, about a minute had passed, and I heard, then saw a truck racing up Faulkner Ave, going north." Vinnie pointed in that direction in case Detective Simon was unaware of her location. He continued, "I didn't think anything of it because someone is always speeding down these streets. Shortly after the truck passed, I heard a screeching of tires more from a sudden stop instead of a squealing sound when accelerating. Again, I didn't think anything of it because, as I said, the park attracts people for various reasons. Could have been kids speeding and suddenly stopping; could have been someone late for work; could have been someone that missed a turn and came to a quick stop trying to make the turn."

"Could have been someone that hit a person on a bike," Detective Simon said as more of a statement than a question. "Could you describe the truck, Mr. Calabrese?"

"It was black or maybe dark blue. Not one of those big full-size ones but a shorter one, with a front and a back seat, you know, four doors. I didn't get the make or model, but it did look fairly new."

"Like that one over there?" Rhonda pointed to a newer model black Honda Ridgeline.

"Well, actually, that is my truck," Vinnie said casually. "Yes, I guess something like mine."

Considering that he had a similar truck to the one he just described, Detective Simon was a bit surprised. Most people, especially innocent ones, would have probably used their vehicle as a point of comparison. It was just more straightforward.

"Ok, Mr. Calabrese, is there anything else you can remember? How many people did you see in the truck? Color of their skin, age, male, female?"

"I think, just a driver, but the car had tinted windows, and it was moving pretty fast, so there is not much more I can tell you. Do you think we are done here?" Vinnie said, showing a lot more anxiousness than he had previously.

"Yeah, we're done. I just need to get your address for our records. Are you going back to fish?"

"No, fishing was slow, and I planned to leave when all this happened. Can you tell me anything about the bike rider?"

"All I can tell you is he was a young male, white, 25, but I can't tell you his name until we notify his relatives," Detective Simon said, closing her notebook. "He was in pretty bad shape. I don't know if he will survive."

"I understand. Tragic that a young person might die on such a nice morning, keeping to themselves, enjoying life," Vinnie said solemnly.

"Yes, it is," Detective Simon added, knowing people are taken from this earth, in tragic or senseless ways, morning, noon, and night whether it was a beautiful day or not. "We did notice he was an organ donor. So, if he, unfortunately, does die, perhaps his lost life will save another," she said while pointing to the hospital complex beyond the trees, knowing he was headed there.

"That seems like a gruesome and uncaring thing to say, Detective."

"I am in the gruesome and uncaring business, sir," Detective Simon said curtly.

Sensing a bit of anger in Detective Simon, he began walking with her to his truck, thinking about his conversation with Frank the previous evening. Vinnie changed the subject and asked, "Do you know anything about organ donors and how long the organs survive after death?"

"Well, that's not part of my job description. I think Doctors try and harvest what they can, but it all depends upon the organ and how long the victim was deceased," Detective Simon said, still somewhat agitated by these questions.

Vinnie started to put his fishing equipment in the bed of his truck, and as he did, Detective Simon strolled around the vehicle, looking for any signs of it being scrapped or dented. No luck. It was too muddy to get a clear look at anything. Detective Simon handed Vinnie her card, thanked him, and told him to call her if he remembered anything else about the incident.

CHAPTER 15

Brooke MacIntosh's team was on alert for a possible lung organ donor. White male, 5'8", 165 lbs., 25 years of age, O positive blood type. Significant trauma was caused by being hit by a car while bike riding. He agreed to be an organ donor through the DMV, and his parents were notified and at the hospital. Brooke had been given a notice by the UNOS database of the potential recipients on her floor. If this man's lungs were harvestable, Brooke knew who would have the highest match rate for this young man's lungs. Brooke thought about all the possible recipients, hoping one on her floor would be the perfect match. Then, as she always did, she thought about the donor. Twenty-five years old, a few years younger than Brooke. He was probably getting some morning exercise riding his bike, something Brooke had done a hundred times in Forest Park. He was trying to stay healthy in the morning and was now dying in the afternoon. Brooke sometimes wondered about the power of God. Although religious, but with some doubt, she often wondered about God's plan for all of us. Was there even a plan?

This process was Brooke's normal progression when a donor was identified. First, compassion for them or their family. Then, questioning the randomness of God's plan. Then, the joy of telling a recipient on her floor that their lucky number had come up. Then, waiting for the donor's death, harvesting the organs, prepping the recipients, and the operation.

Finally, the crossing of fingers for a full recovery. While the UNOS national donor database matched those who became donors with those who were recipients, the match criteria were impersonal. Blood type, body size, location of organ compared to the recipient. There were no names, backstories, or mention of the need or value of the person getting the organ, although pediatric transplants did have some priority. It was so impersonal, but Brooke knew and cared for her patients. Brook knew their stories. She knew what type of life they lived and what their future held. As she thought about it, she began to think about Dr. Finnegan's seminar, bringing the donor and recipient together to improve the outcome hopefully.

Perhaps he was correct that the organs donated carried the donor's spirit into the recipient's body. After all, an organ was a living tissue. If a heavy drinker donated their liver to a non-drinker, would the history of that liver carry on with the new recipient? Would the organ and the recipient do better if, before the transplant happened, there was some connection between both people?

Brooke knew that the transplant process had improved in leaps and bounds over the years, and more people were getting and surviving transplants. But she also understood so many people needing transplants never got them because of the matching process. She also knew those fortunate to match were not all fortunate post-transplant, as some died or rejected the organ. Thinking about all this made her head spin, and she needed to shake away the fog in her brain and concentrate on the patient soon to receive the donor's organs. Brooke looked forward to clearing her mind and taking a run in the park as soon as her shift ended.

CHAPTER 16

Detective Simon was one of the first officials to be notified that Brian Coffman, the hit and run victim in Forest Park, had died. Initially, hit and runs are considered vehicular manslaughter, but until Detective Simon could find the driver, she could not rule out any motive. She looked at her notes from that morning, including her talk with Vinnie Calabrese, and decided to run his plates to be sure he was clean. Putting his name in the database, nothing unusual came up. The vehicle, a 2019 Honda Ridgeline pick-up truck, was leased and had no evidence of an insurance claim or a parking ticket issued against it in the two years Vinnie owned it. She looked further into Vinnie's history with his insurance company and the DMV and found that outside of a few speeding tickets over the years, Mr. Calabrese's record was clean.

She sighed and realized she would have to add Brian Coffman's investigation into her already backlogged cases. While she had a sense of indifference in solving drug-related murders, she had a sense of urgency, maybe sympathy, in solving Brian Coffman's death. His death could've been murder, but it was probably an accident. While not sure she believed it, she vowed to herself to devote the energies necessary to solve all the crimes, regardless of the victim, now stored in the files on her computer.

Clicking on her laptop files, she knew what a difficult task she had in front of her. William Burroughs was still dead. The case was still unsolved, and there were still no promising leads. She paged through her notes and listened again to some of the "tips" that came in through the St. Louis police anonymous hotline. Most of the leads and tips were street gossip or revenge tips pointing the finger at suspects who could not possibly be tied to the crime. Nothing jumped out except one.

Someone had mentioned that about 30 minutes before William Burrough's killing, a newer white Audi A6 or A8 parked, and two young black males exited the vehicle.

After everyone had fled the house, the two males got in the white Audi and drove off. The tipster did not identify the license plates, and no further description of the males or the driver was on the tip line. The tipster noted that the driver stayed in the car. This information seemed important, but since it was anonymous, there was no one Detective Simon could follow up with and ask more questions. Before drawing any conclusions, she needed to think about this for a bit, but she hoped the white Audi and its occupants would appear again at another crime scene.

She clicked on another file: the overdose victim found near Pappy's BBQ on Olive. The victim had a license identifying him as Tayjon Reynolds, Black, age 32, 5' 9", 160 lbs. Cause of death: heroin overdose, not the gruesome removal of the man's kidney. No eyewitnesses. No tips on the anonymous hotline. The only odd thing that stood out on the report was after the next of kin was notified, they asked that the body be brought not to the morgue but to a business called Arch City Transplant Center. Since Simon did not care about the body after death, she ignored that piece of information. But since the crime had occurred in a parking lot of a Budget Rental Car location and across from Pappy's, one of the area's most popular restaurants, she knew there would be surveillance cameras all over the businesses and on the streets. The location was just east of the St. Louis University campus, and while the neighborhood was reasonably safe during the day, it had its share of criminal activity at night. So, there were plenty of cameras, and since it was lunchtime, there was no better reason to visit Pappy's for surveillance camera footage to review and maybe some BBQ afterward.

Driving to Pappy's, she planned to look at the footage and then hopefully eat. Maybe if she were lucky, they would slide her a plate of baby back ribs while she was viewing the footage. Settling in the manager's office, she pulled up video, and zeroing in within one hour before they found the body, she saw what looked like the victim crossing the street from Pappy's parking lot to the Budget parking lot. She also wanted to look at the interior camera footage to see if Mr. Reynolds had a little BBQ before he decided to shoot up. *That would be a waste of a good BBQ on a junkie,* she thought to herself. After reviewing the street cameras and determining that Mr. Reynolds walked from the vicinity of Pappy's to the Budget parking lot, she reviewed interior footage. Mr. Reynolds did not seem to have made BBQ his last meal, as he was not on any interior footage. The smell of BBQ and her hunger pains were getting to her. She knew she had to do two more things: eat and look at the Budget Car camera footage. Before she could go to Budget, a server came up to the office with a full plate of ribs, beans, coleslaw, and apple sauce, to her surprise and enjoyment.

"Enjoy, Detective," the young woman said with a smile. "Thanks for keeping the streets safe." While Detective Simon never asked for a free meal, and because she was usually in plain clothes, she rarely got offered one. Her plan to look at footage first resulted in a delicious yet messy plate of ribs. As she dug in, she realized how messy they would be to eat. So, she turned off the camera playback equipment so as not to smear it with BBQ sauce.

Had she waited a few minutes before eating or been slightly sloppy while eating, she would have seen footage of a newer model white Audi sedan leaving the parking lot behind Pappy's and heading east on Olive past the Budget parking lot.

CHAPTER 17

Her shift was over, and Brooke changed into running clothes heading west from the hospital for a run in the park. She was going to take it easy today and needed the run more to clear her head than for maximum exertion. Brooke ran track in high school, and her speed and stamina only improved over time. While younger, she ran to compete but now ran to keep herself in excellent physical and mental shape. When Brooke wanted a more leisurely run, she stuck to the inner paths of the park as they took her past a variety of the park's architecture, flora, fauna, and attractions.

It was a beautiful day, and Brooke wanted to see what was blooming in the gardens and playing at the Muny this summer, so she headed in that direction. As she was running, she noticed a man behind her hurrying his pace as if to catch her. Even though he did not look dangerous, Brooke was in no mood to be hit on while running, an experience that happened way too often during her runs but one Brooke knew how to handle. Brooke decided to shake this guy. It was best to hit some hills, and she took one of the highest ones to the World's Fair Pavilion on Government Hill, the highest point in the park and a reminder of the breathtaking view fair goers must have had in 1904. The first part of the climb was the hill, and most unwelcome admirers may try to follow her up, but the second part was stairs, where most men would give up. As she reached the top, she turned and saw the man she assumed was following her turn back down, probably realizing it was not worth a heart attack to just be rejected by her. When she thought it was safe, she ran back down the hill to the Boat House to grab a bottle of water and to cool down. She then walked from the Boathouse to the Muny Theater box office to see what was playing that evening and later in the summer. As she was reading about the upcoming plays and times, she did not notice a man sidling up to her.

"My parents took me here when I was young, and I have loved it ever since," said the man to no one in particular. Looking over to see if maybe he was talking to someone, Brooke realized he was talking to her, and as she turned, he asked, "What is your favorite play?"

"Hmm," Brooke stammered, not sure if she wanted to engage in a conversation with a stranger, but she instead said, "Well, my parents first took me to see "Mary Poppins" when I was 11, but my favorite play is "Sound of Music." I love any Rodgers and Hammerstein musical."

"And running, I take it?" he said back to her, moving on from the arts portion of this conversation.

"Yeah, and running, and that is what I should be doing," Brooke said as she quickly sipped the last of her water to emphasize that it was time to go. But something about this man stopped her.

"Do I know you?" she asked. "You look familiar."

"Well, not to freak you out, but I was the guy trying unsuccessfully to catch up to you. You put me in my place with that burst up Government Hill," he said.

Creep was the first thought Brooke had, but she knew she was safe with other visitors crowding the area nearby. Besides, she knew she could outrun him if needed, so she stayed reasonably calm.

"Well, although I am not in your league, I frequently run in the park. So, if you recognize me, perhaps our paths have crossed," he laughed.

Recognition came to Brooke's face slowly, not from knowing him as a fellow runner or maybe today's stalker, but as he took off his ball cap to wipe the sweat from his face, she began to smile and relax. "Well, perhaps, but I think our paths crossed at the transplant seminar you spoke at last week. You're Dr. Finnegan?" She asked not as much as a question but as an affirmation.

"Guilty as charged," he laughed. "Though I prefer the less formal Alex, here on the streets. After all, Doctor seems a bit formal when you wear running clothes and sweat like a pig."

"Brooke MacIntosh, Dr. Finnegan," she said, wiping her hand on her skintight Lulu Lemon's, then extending it to him. "I am a nurse at Barnes, and it is always a bit disrespectful to call a doctor by his first name."

"Fair enough, Brooke. So, what was your interest in the transplant seminar?"

"I am one of the transplant coordinators at Barnes, and I was attending to improve my knowledge on the changes in the industry."

"And did you? Improve your knowledge?" he asked, knowing what the answer would be.

"More than improved it. The seminar awakened my mind to new possibilities in organ transplantation that I never knew existed; capped off, I must say, by your finale," Brooke said. She instantly regretted that she spoke so enthusiastically, sounding like someone with a schoolyard crush on the man standing next to her.

Brooke looked at her Apple watch, trying to hide her embarrassment while also checking on the lateness of the day. She slowly started light stretches, indicating it was time to limber up and finish her run.

Sensing she was about to leave, Alex quickly added, "Well, if the seminar awakened your mind, no telling what a tour of my facility would do for you. Why don't you stop by some time, and I will give you some insight beyond what I could or wanted to cover at the seminar?"

"Really?" Brooke said again with a little more schoolgirl crush than intended. "That would be great. I will take you up on that and thank you for the offer." Then to fill an awkward silence, she added, "Well, I need to run and head back to Barnes."

"Alright. I am going the other way. I still have time to do another lap around the park maybe," he said, not with any hint of boasting, just spoke as a matter of fact.

As Brooke began to stroll away, she turned and yelled back, "Oh, and by the way, Young Frankenstein is one of my favorite movies, as well." She did not know if he heard her as he did not turn around, but she did not feel dumb saying it, instead feeling something else, a jolt of energy and a feeling of lightness that made the last two miles of her run go by effortlessly.

CHAPTER 18

As he was cooking dinner, Vinnie looked down at his phone and noticed a text from Ellen. It read: "Check out the 6:00 p.m. local news on KSDK today. You might see yours truly." ☺

Not usually a news watcher, Vinnie checked the time on his phone. Noticing it was almost 6:00, he turned on the TV and planned to catch the news while he ate. Living on his own for the last two years, most of his meals were spent eating alone, usually watching a game or old movie. Tonight, he would indulge Ellen and watch the news.

Ten minutes into the newscast, the announcer, Jennifer Jackson, came back from the commercial and introduced her newest segment.

"Giving life when death seems so close. St. Louis' doctors are changing how we think about transplants."

Listening now more intently, Vinnie soon noticed Dr. Alex Finnegan appearing on screen, talking about his vision and their work at Arch City Transplants. He quickly looked for his remote control to turn the volume up. While he had little interest in what Finnegan had to say, he listened for a few more minutes. He was rewarded as the interviewer then turned and introduced Dr. Ellen James-Calabrese, Chief Medical Officer, to get her opinion on The Center and its vision.

Well, that was nice, he thought. That ego manic, Finnegan, shared the limelight with Ellen for a few minutes. Probably because the newscaster was female and she wanted Ellen's viewpoint, Vinnie thought cynically. The five-minute segment ended with a brief video overview of The Center's facilities and then another commercial break.

Vinnie looked down at his phone and texted Ellen, "I caught your segment on TV. Congrats." After a brief pause, he added, "You looked good." ☺

Putting his phone aside while cleaning up dinner, it buzzed about five minutes later.

"Good enough to take me to dinner?" ☺

Despite that Vinnie had just eaten, he texted back: "Lorenzo's at 7:30?"

"See you there," she pinged back, almost too quickly. Vinnie's customary cynicism gave way to a bit of excitement.

Since Lorenzos was only a few blocks from Vinnie's home, he, of course, would walk. He left early, though, thinking he would take a few extra blocks around his neighborhood to work off the meal he had just finished.

He did not know why, but he did not want Ellen to know he had already eaten when he accepted her invitation. If she did, he thought it would seem like he was needy or lonely. He was, but he did not want or need sympathy from Ellen. He knew it would not be too difficult to eat anything on Lorenzo's menu, which featured Northern Italian recipes. So, he knew a little walk would help the digestive system help him conceal the fact that he had already eaten and allow him to eat some more.

During his 45-minute stroll around his neighborhood, Vinnie tossed a few coins for good luck into the Piazza Imo Fountain across from St. Ambrose Church. He then peeked into the Bocce Ball courts at Milo's to see if any old friends were playing or drinking. They weren't. He finally reached Lorenzo's and grabbed a seat at the bar to wait for Ellen. After ordering his usual Tito's Vodka Martini - straight up with blue cheese olives, he perused the menu, which he knew by memory, and at 7:30 on the dot, in walked Ellen. They had their choice of tables as it was not crowded, so Vinnie picked a corner table. After countless times eating there with

Ellen, he knew not to grab the bench seat tables where someone looked at the wall while the other person looked at the diners in the restaurant.

Because Vinnie or Ellen never wanted to face the wall, they would sit on one side as a couple. Ellen always thought it made them look like teenagers, but Vinnie always enjoyed seated side by side, and as his hearing diminished, he liked it because he could hear what Ellen was saying.

As soon as the hostess removed the two extra place settings, Vinnie quickly blurted out, "I am glad that jerk let you talk."

Without commenting, Ellen looked at Vinnie, then at his nearly empty martini glass, and said, "How many of those have you had?"

"Just this one, so far, but I always could use a drinking companion," Vinnie said, failing to mention the two glasses of wine he had at home. Their waiter appeared and asked for Ellen's drink order.

"I will have a Cosmo," she said, turning to the waiter, "And please bring some menus. I am famished."

Shortly after perusing the menus, Ellen ordered the Barramundi; a Mediterranean white fish served over a bed of risotto. Although still full of his meal two hours ago, Vinnie chose the Chicken Spiedini stuffed with spinach and prosciutto. Not a lite meal but one of Vinnie's favorites.

As the waiter brought Ellen's drink, she asked Vinnie, "So, what did you think of the segment?"

"To be honest, I am not sure I understood it all that well," Vinnie replied, even though it was more so that he did not listen to the news story versus understanding it.

"What didn't you understand?" Ellen asked. Without waiting for Vinnie's reply, she continued, "We are trying to change the way society views life and death choices, as well as how a donor and the recipient are prepared, in many cases, before needing a transplant. We believe that eliminating the time lag between a donor's death and when the organ is transplanted will increase our success rate. We believe an organ carries the deceased person's life into the recipient's body. Our goal is to foster that transportation of life, which is really what a transplant is."

Had Vinnie listened to the segment on the news, he would have realized Ellen had just repeated the same talking points as on TV. Rather than respond, ask a question, or show the faintest interest in what Ellen just said, all he could muster was a slightly slurred, "So, why did you want to meet me for dinner?"

Ellen, feeling the familiar rise of frustration with Vinnie not really listening to her, or showing any interest in her work, curtly replied, "Well, I was hungry, you were close by, and I did not want to eat alone. Are you happy?"

Vinnie, sensing the evening was about to take a turn in the wrong direction from what his mind had conjured up earlier, turned the tide by asking, "So, what are the greatest obstacles to the Transplant Center achieving its goals? Is it being accepted by the medical industry? Is it the willingness of donors and recipients to try this innovative approach? Or, and he couldn't stop himself, "is it finding someone to play Dr. Frankenstein...I mean, Dr. Finnegan, when the movie comes out?"

Ellen could not hold back her laughter after that comment and her quiet satisfaction that perhaps Vinnie was listening to her and interested in her work. "Well," she said with a slight grin, "because Alex is so handsome," pausing briefly to return the jab, "I think Matthew McConaughey or Patrick Dempsey would be a perfect Dr. Frankenstein, but I am not sure who I want to play me? Should it be Robin Wright or Laura Linney?"

"Definitely Robin Wright," said Vinnie. "And let's toast to that with two more drinks," signaling to the waiter and silently smiling as maybe the dinner had begun to turn back his way.

CHAPTER 19

Frank Esposito was struggling, both physically and mentally. He was unsure, which was taking a heavier toll on him and his family. After his initial diagnosis, Frank sat his family down. He explained what Dr. Spiros had told him the best he could to his three sons and wife, Sue. It hit them all hard, beyond the thought of possibly losing Frank to this illness and the continued string of lousy news Frank experienced in life. If there was a poster with the caption "Why do bad things happen to good people?" Frank Esposito's photo would be on it. But offsetting the bad news, of which Frank seemed always to get a disproportionate share, was Frank's incredible optimism and cheerful attitude regardless of what fate delivered. Frank's family fed off Frank's optimism and always believed they could overcome anything thrown at them in life. They would handle this like they handled everything: prayers and faith in each other.

It had been two months since his diagnosis, and he was shocked at how quickly the disease progressed and how poorly he felt. He knew he had to improve his health to be in better shape to receive a lung transplant, a conclusion Frank now readily admitted was his only chance to survive, but he could barely get off the couch long enough to exercise. He slept on the couch, sitting up. If he laid down at any point, it would create a series of violent coughing attacks.

It would take him about two hours to take a shower. He also needed to lose 30 pounds and build up his endurance.

At first, he used a secondhand treadmill at home that his brother-in-law, Vinnie, had brought over, but then he started rehab at the hospital so his Doctor could more closely monitor him. His breathing became more difficult. His home, rooms once filled with his grandkids' toys, were now filled with oxygen cylinders he was going through at a rate of four a day.

Frank was an eternal optimist, but it seemed like he was in a three-legged race. His body was competing to get sick enough to be eligible for a transplant while healthy enough to accept a transplant, and finally hoping the first two outcomes would beat the last one to the finish line, death from the disease.

Chapter 20

❧

Brooke arrived at the Arch City Transplant Center at 10:00 a.m. for her facility tour. The Center was on Laclede and Taylor, east of the extensive medical complexes of Barnes and the St. Louis Children's Hospitals and the medical school facilities associated with Washington University. Brooke did not know what to expect when she arrived, but when she did, her initial surprise was the lobby seemed less like a medical facility and more like a luxury living center. She double-checked the address to make sure she was in the correct building.

To Brooke's surprise, the receptionist greeted her and already had a packet of information and a visitor ID prepared. She mentioned that Dr. Finnegan would be joining her at some point, but the Tour Coordinator, Molly, would be down shortly to start the tour. Brooke sat in a very modern yet comfortable chair while she waited and perused the information in the packet. She was slightly disappointed that Dr. Finnegan was not there to greet her but thought how silly it was of her to think he would have time to spend hours with her. She felt sillier when she looked down at her outfit, knowing it was the final selection of ten she had tried that morning. Brooke wanted to achieve the perfect balance of professionalism and style with maybe a little sexiness. She chose a fitted jacket, black pencil skirt, and open towed pumps with heels slightly higher and much more uncomfortable than she usually would wear during the day. Brooke did remember Dr. Finnegan spending a few lingering seconds staring at her body during their encounter at the park. Because of that, she thought a slight dash of sexiness was appropriate. Brooke was an intelligent woman but still in a man's world, and she assumed that Dr. Finnegan had perhaps additional reasons to ask her to tour the facility. Well, two could play that game. Now though, she thought it made no sense, and she had wished she had just come over in her everyday work clothes of scrubs and comfortable running shoes.

But as soon as her tour coordinator Molly came into view, Brooke was glad she did not wear scrubs as Molly looked more like a model coming down the runway than a tour coordinator at a medical facility. Molly, tall with an athletic physique, greeted Brooke. She had a dazzling smile of the whitest teeth Brooke had ever seen, framed by a perfect face and long auburn hair. She extended her hand to Brooke, saying with a faint southern accent, "Brooke, it is so nice to meet you, and welcome to The Arch City Transplant Center. Dr. Finnegan wanted me to let you know how sorry he is that he could not greet you upon arrival, but a bit of an emergency came up, and he will join us shortly."

"Pleasure to meet you, Molly. I am sure Dr. Finnegan is very busy, and if he even stops by to say hello, that is fine with me. I would not expect someone as busy as he is to be able to spend much time doing a facility tour."

"You are getting the VIP tour, Brooke, not the standard facility tour. Only Dr. Finnegan gives the VIP tours," she said with a wry smile, or at least Brooke thought she detected one.

As they walked, Molly began with an overview of The Center, providing its history, size, square footage, staff and patients, and the number of successful transplants it has handled since opening last year. She stopped in front of a wall of photos described as "Our Heroes" depicting the donor and the organ recipient, organized by type of transplant.

The photos and information were inconsistent; in some cases, information on both the donor and recipient, including names, was listed. In other cases, both images were there, but no names were listed, and finally, only the recipient was listed, not the donor.

Sensing Brooke's question before she could ask it, Molly, with a practiced speech, said, "As you can see, the information is not consistent. However, look at the progression of time. You will see that the longer The Center has been open, the more people are comfortable sharing their part in our vision of making transplantation a celebration of joined lives going forward due to organ donation. As you know, Brooke, the transplant industry has been traditionally cloaked in anonymity; whose organs are used, who gets one, what the criteria are, but we hope to change all that with The Center's work."

Walking as she talked, Molly said, "Sorry to rush you along, but we have a lot to see before you meet with Dr. Finnegan before lunch. You can join him for lunch, can't you?"

As they waited for the elevator to take them to the upper floors of The Center, Brooke asked, "Molly, how long have you been giving tours?"

"Well, I have been only doing tours for the last three months. I got the job right after starting medical school at Wash U. I'm a first-year."

"Oh, congratulations," Brooke said. "That must be hard balancing medical school with a job?"

"Well, it's only part-time, and many of us here are in medical school. We have a schedule that coordinates the time we need for classroom and clinicals and the time needed here. Dr. Finnegan, and Dr. Calabrese, our Chief Medical Officer, work very closely with the school to ensure we get the proper balance, and we also learn so much here. Dr. Finnegan is a Wash U graduate, and I know he's a huge donor to the school, so it all seems to work out."

The elevator chimed, indicating the door opening, and two young women, who seemed to be clones of Molly, exited. Molly introduced them quickly, saying, "Brooke, this is Lauren and Elizabeth, classmates of mine who also work at The Center." With no time for longer pleasantries, Brooke smiled, said hi, and the elevator doors closed, taking Molly and her up to the second floor.

Once on the second floor, Molly explained what they were to see. "There are five main areas to The Center. Two, which I will call the non-clinical areas, are on this floor. The clinical areas, including the organ prep and operating suites, are on the 3rd floor, and our technology center, which makes everything work, is on the 4th floor, as are the executive offices and dining room. I believe Dr. Finnegan will meet you on the 4th floor, and you can decide whether to eat lunch before or after visiting the organ prep and operating suites."

An operating room is not gory as a layperson might think. It is antiseptic, sterile, and a very controlled environment, usually tranquil with the Doctor's choice of music playing. She had seen many operations, so nothing going on there would bother Brooke. Nor would the organ prep area, a morgue of sorts, where she assumed the organs were removed as soon as the donor passed. Brooke had seen plenty of death and understood it as part of the life circle. She thought Molly was a bit naïve to believe that anything she saw at the Transplant Center would bother her and categorized Molly's comments as a typical first-year medical student. So smug that they are in medical school and already demeaning nurses as beneath them. Molly would learn to appreciate nurses as all doctors do. Nurses make the Doctor's job easy by dealing with the crap they did not want or could do. After all, Brooke knew that when a patient is in the hospital, it is the nurses whose name they call. It's the nurse's comfort that patients want and need, which is not always a given by doctors.

Perhaps sensing she misspoke, Molly covered herself by saying, "Well, of course, Brooke, in your job, I am sure you have seen everything, and nothing you will see here will bother you."

Continuing down the hall with only the clicking of their heels, breaking the now uncomfortable silence, Molly entered a double door that led to a lobby divided into two sections and explained what they were seeing.

"This is our transitional living area. If it helps you visualize, think of this in terms of independent living, assisted living, nursing home, and hospice and the stages one goes through as one ages. On the left side is the living area of those patients who are terminal and who have agreed to provide their organs when they pass. Within this area are stages of transition that the patient goes through as they move on to death, each stage designed for their comfort. The area on the right is the living area for those patients who will be recipients of the organs. Again, their living area moves them through the stages of preparing to get an organ. In some cases, their living area is like home. Then as we prepare them for a transplant, they move to a more medical setting where we can monitor their vitals and prepare them for surgery. There is a common or shared area where patients, donors, recipients, and their families can meet and learn about each other, an important part of our vision that we believe helps in the success of the transplant."

"Can we go in?" Brooke asked.

"Of course. I hate to use the phrase: *'this is what sells the concept,'* but in many cases, it does. You must see how the patients interact with each other. Showing both donor and recipient, and their families, how an organ donation bonds both groups of people, helps them accept what is about to happen in the most positive way possible."

"But there is so much regulation regarding transplants. There are priority lists based on need and match. How does The Center get around or work within the law?" Brooke asked with a bit of puzzlement on her face.

"Probably a better question for Dr. Finnegan, Brooke."

Molly then used the key card to open the second set of double doors, leading down a corridor flanked by nicely appointed hotel rooms with hospital beds. As they walked down the hall, Molly mentioned that they had permission to meet with both a donor and a recipient and their families.

"We will meet the Johnson and Ortel families in our shared family area. Feel free to ask them any questions you may have."

Entering a large room with sunlight shining through floor-to-ceiling windows, Brooke encountered a small group of people comfortably sitting in a living room setting, watching a large TV that played what looked to be old home videos.

"Sorry to disturb everyone," Molly said. "This is Brooke MacIntosh, a special guest of Dr. Finnegan's, and if we could take some time to let her meet you all and ask some questions, that would be great."

A woman, who looked to be about 45, turned down the volume on the TV and then turned to Brooke.

"Hello, Brooke. So nice to meet you. Sorry for the TV being so loud, but when you have several of us hard of hearing, we tend to have the volume a little louder than we should. I am Nancy Johnson, and this is my sister, Marianne, and her husband, Bill. Over there on the couch is our father, Sam Johnson."

Brooke quickly scanned all the people as she introduced them but could not ascertain that Sam Johnson, who looked to be around 70, was the future donor or recipient.

Nancy continued, "I will let Peggy Ortel introduce her clan." Another woman, perhaps a little older than Nancy, said, "Hi, Brooke. I am Peggy Ortel, and this is my husband, Chuck, and our sons Wyatt and Wesley."

"Please take a seat," Peggy said. "We like to play a little game to break the ice when we have a visitors tour."

Brooke took a seat, as did Molly. "Well, Molly knows the answers, so she can't play, but we like to ask visitors who is the donor and recipient?"

"Hmm, hmm," Brooke stalled, as she knew any answer was probably wrong and might upset some family members. "I really couldn't say."

With that, several members of both families laughed, and Peggy said, "Hah, no one ever wants to answer that question. Our visitors are so uncomfortable even touring that answering such a private question usually gets that response."

"But to put your mind at ease, Brooke," Nancy interjected, "Sam, my father is the donor, and Chuck, Peggy's husband, is the recipient."

"Oh, I am so sorry, Nancy."

"Thank you, Brooke. It's ok. We have all shed a million tears, but getting to know Peggy's family and Chuck especially, has made what we know is the inevitable a little more acceptable."

Molly jumped in part because she knew both families had more of the story and would spend hours if you left them to tell it. Plus, she was trying to keep a schedule per Dr. Finnegan, who always encouraged tours but balanced them with the privacy of each family.

"Nancy, Peggy, or anybody, why don't you tell Brooke what you are doing here today."

Sam Johnson surprisingly piped up a little more strongly and loudly than Brooke expected. "I will tell you what the hell we are doing here. We are making sure that my heart is going to a good place. We are making sure Chuck can handle carrying around my big heart because you know he has a weak one. I was in the Marines, and Chuck was in the Navy. You know those Navy boys could never carry the water for a marine."

Laughter again from everyone, but Brooke could see a bit of sadness in the eyes of a few of the family members.

When the laughter subsided, Nancy said, "You caught us watching some old family videos of both families. Getting to know our history and what makes us click. It gives us peace knowing that when my dad passes, his heart is going to a man who shares his values and whose family matters to him."

"Well, I am giving some of my other organs up, too," Sam yelled out, "but who gets my heart is what matters. Despite being in the Navy, Chuck is a good man, and I hope my heart helps him enjoy more time with his grandkids."

"Damn it, Sam. You, old leather neck. You always make me cry. Stop it," Chuck quietly said, now joined in tears by his two sons.

Sam chimed in, "Maybe my heart will toughen you up, Navy boy."

Brooke sensed it was time to leave these families, and while she had hundreds of questions, she did not want to overstay her welcome. And besides, she was having trouble fighting back her tears, an emotion that she did a good job hiding when dealing with her patients.

As they left the unit and headed up to the fourth floor, Molly told Brooke that the family visit part of the tour was always gut-wrenching, saying the visitors always had a tough time absorbing what was happening. Usually, The Center picked out families that had gotten to know each other quite well, and the grief and guilt were gone for the time being.

"How much time do Mr. Johnson and Mr. Ortel have?" Brooke asked. Before Molly could answer that question, the elevator door opened, and in it, Dr. Finnegan.

"Hello Brooke, hello Molly," Dr. Finnegan said with a tone and enthusiasm more lighthearted than Brooke was feeling now.

As a bit of explanation, Molly said, "We just got done visiting with the Johnson and Ortel families."

"Oh. That is always tough," Dr. Finnegan said more somberly. "Good people. Hopefully, Brooke, you will see that what we are doing here makes this reality more tolerable to all families." The elevator opened to the 4th floor, and Dr. Finnegan said to Molly, "Thank you, dear. I will take it from here." I hope the first semester is going well for you?"

"All good, Doctor," Molly replied, waving bye as the elevator door closed on her, leaving Brooke and Dr. Finnegan in the lobby of the very luxurious executive offices.

Looking at his watch and seeing it was nearly noon, and without really asking, Dr. Finnegan said, "I am sure you have lots of questions. Let's get you off those shoes for an hour and cover your questions over lunch."

"That sounds great, Dr. Finnegan," replied Brooke, though she thought that was an odd way to describe a lunch invitation by noticing her shoes. But she had so many questions that she was almost dizzy with them swirling around in her brain.

"I assume Molly mentioned that our Chief Medical Officer, Dr. Ellen James-Calabrese, will join us for lunch. Is that ok, Brooke?"

"Certainly," she said as they both entered a small but comfortable private dining room with several white-clothed tables with settings for four or two people. Sitting at one of the tables was a very stylish woman who stood up to greet them. She said, "Hi, Brooke. I am Dr. Ellen James-Calabrese."

"Pleasure to meet you, Dr. Calabrese," Brooke said, extending her hand.

"Please call me Ellen."

Before Brooke could answer, Dr. Finnegan interjected, "I tried Ellen, but she has been taught well and only will address me, and I assume you too, as Doctor. But perhaps someday, if she sees us as colleagues, she will call us by our first name."

Colleagues? Second odd comment, thought Brooke. She just sat down and smiled, happy to get off her feet, as she was not used to wearing heels.

After settling in and making small talk while a waiter took their drink order, which was ice tea for everyone, Dr. Calabrese asked Brooke how the tour had been so far.

"It's been good. Very informative and not what I expected, but I was not sure what to expect, to be honest with you."

"How so?" Dr. Finnegan asked.

"Well, I thought it was going to be more of a clinical or health care setting, and from what I have seen so far, it seemed more like an upscale assisted living center."

"Good. That's what we want our visitors to see. Of course, you will see some of the more clinical and medical operations you would expect us to have in The Center after lunch. We don't take prospective donors or recipients into the medical or surgical side of the business. I think it would become too real for them, but we will show that to you because it is important."

"Thank you both for taking time in your day to give me such an exhaustive tour, but if you are busy, I don't have to see all of that. And I know you are busy," Brooke politely said.

Dr. Calabrese then chimed in, "Well, Brooke, you must leave here understanding what we are trying to accomplish and how we plan to accomplish it. A person in your position, in most likelihood, will interact with us, hopefully, advocate for us, or maybe down the road, even work with us. We are a growing and dynamic company after all."

The conversation seemed to be taking a turn beyond what Brooke had expected. It was not necessarily a negative turn, as Brooke was savvy enough to always keep her eye out for opportunities to keep growing professionally. She knew associations with accomplished medical professionals and business visionaries were critical to her career.

After ordering, Dr. Calabrese changed subjects and asked Brooke about her educational background, her work experience, and in a very delicate way, some personal questions. Brooke was getting the sense that Dr. Calabrese was interviewing her, a thought that was not unfounded as Dr. Calabrese prefaced her questions by saying: "Brooke, I know this seems like an interview but tell us a bit about yourself while we wait for our food to arrive."

Brooke went through her education experience, describing her undergrad and master's degree attainment at St. Louis University. She talked about her initial jobs at St. Louis University Hospital in the ER, then her move to Barnes, where she started in the ICU and was now a transplant coordinator on the pulmonary floor. She sidestepped the personal question only to say she was born and raised in Kirkwood and now lived in the Lafayette Square neighborhood. That was enough personal information. Brooke felt that Ellen already knew all about her, perhaps even more than she was letting on.

Dr. Calabrese, who always liked to keep everyone on their toes, was not going to let Brooke get a pass on personal questions. She asked if she was related to the people who owned MacIntosh's restaurant. Brooke acknowledged that, yes, the restaurant is owned by her parents. She shouldn't have been surprised by the question, considering the restaurant was well known locally and had been open for nearly 30 years.

"Oh, I love that restaurant. It used to be my go-to breakfast spot when I lived out that way," Dr. Calabrese added lightly. "I guess you worked there from time to time, as most restaurants are family businesses. Am I right?"

"You are right. I worked, well still work, and help when I can, waitressing and hosting. Anything my mom and dad need me to do."

"That's great, Brooke. It is nice to see young people like yourself work hard for their goals but still help the family. I hope the Covid lockdowns were not too hard on the restaurant?"

"Unfortunately, it has been tough for my parents and some of our employees, but somehow, we will make it," Brooke said while she stirred her spoon in her bowl of soup which had been untouched and was now cold.

Sensing it was time to move on, Dr. Calabrese turned to Dr. Finnegan and asked, "Alex, why don't you give Brooke an overview of what she will see next."

Throughout the entire back and forth between Dr. Calabrese and Brooke, Dr. Finnegan was silent or was focused on finishing his lunch, which now Brooke wished she had, as she had barely eaten anything, and her energy level was dropping.

"Brooke, the best part of our tour is you get to take a breather from Ellen's interrogation of you. Ellen is relentless, and we are all afraid of her," Dr. Finnegan said with mock fear as he looked up at Ellen to get her reaction.

Ellen added, "Alex, you know I interrogate our guests so that you can eat because I know what a grouch you can be if you don't eat."

Turning to Brooke, "I am sorry if I was rapid firing in-your-face questions. It is the trait my ex-husband hated most about me, but I think it," looking playfully at Dr. Finnegan, "is a trait my 'work husband' likes best about me." She put an exaggerated emphasis with air quotes on 'work husband.'

"So true. As long Ellen doesn't probe me as aggressively as she just did you," Dr. Finnegan laughed.

For a minute, Brooke wondered if the server brought alcohol to both Doctors, and she missed it. Their mood and banter instantly became playful and cheerful, or perhaps there was something more personal between them?

Bringing her back to reality, Dr. Finnegan got up and said, "Let's go, Brooke. I will show you the guts of the operation, no pun intended, and Ellen will interrogate our next visitor."

With that, Ellen warmly shook Brooke's hand and offered her card, adding, "Brooke, dear, thanks so much for visiting us today, and if there is anything you want to follow up on, please call my cell phone. Also, if you don't mind, I may follow up with you for some additional questions."

"By all means, please feel free to call me and thank you for your time," Brooke replied and then left with Dr. Finnegan.

CHAPTER 21

After exiting the dining room, Dr. Finnegan and Brooke headed down a corridor to a very large room filled with nearly 30 large monitors on the wall. The room was darkly lit with soothing music overhead, occupied by some young men and women working feverishly on their computer screens. As they did, it seemed data and graphs changed on the large monitors.

"This is the GUTS of our operation, Brooke." Brooke thought the word was in bad taste, and she cringed when she heard it.

"I know it is a bad choice of words. But GUTS is an internal acronym, which means 'Get Us Transplants Soon' and describes what The Center is all about. It also describes that what we are doing here, pushing the boundaries of societies' beliefs, also takes some guts. I know it's a little offensive, but one of the computer jocks in here came up with it, and who was I to tell them it is in bad taste? If you look at the folks in this room, I am sure defining taste is not what drives them to get up in the morning. But I promise you we will not be making t-shirts or advertising with that name."

Knowing that computer programmers have a bizarre sense of humor, Brooke said, "Well, despite the weird and distasteful name, it sparks a question lingering in my mind since I went to your seminar and now taking the tour. How do you calibrate what you do here with the transplant regulations and procedures the health care industry and government have followed for years? It seems that you are breaking the rules, jumping the line."

"Good questions which we get all the time from our investors, our patients, health care professionals, lawyers, politicians, and the retched media. And my answer is simple. We follow the rules when they work for all in need, and when they don't, we change them to make them work better. Another way of saying it is that if we can't create enough organ supply, maybe the rules need to be broken. We will work within the current system, but every day we work toward changing the system either through legislation, ingenuity, pushing the envelope, or plain old capitalism."

"Sorry, Dr. Finnegan, that sounds like a bunch of corporate double-speak to me," Brooke said, feeling and sounding a bit feisty as she was probably food-deprived, and it was making her punchy. "You need to explain that."

"Ok, let me walk you through our process. Let's sit in the conference room, though, because it's a lengthy explanation, and I have some visuals that may help."

As they sat in the conference room, Dr. Finnegan went to the white-board and outlined his approach and vision of The Center along with the current state of the transplant industry.

"Ok, Brooke. The transplant process or industry, and it is an industry, by the way, is one controlled by the government, filled with mismanagement, inefficiencies, and probably some corruption. It relies on supply and demand, not unlike any industry. A good analogy is the food business or any business that provides perishable goods and associated spoilage of the product, which in this case are human organs."

Although Brooke cringed as he callously described what she considered something sacred, the passing of organs from one person to another, she could sense that the business side of Dr. Finnegan was speaking to her now, and she sat transfixed by his explanation.

He continued, "Our supply are people who die but have agreed to give their organs upon death. Our demand is for people who need organs. Both the donor and the recipient, as well as the organs, are perishable. The process to improve our yield, so to speak, is to get access to more organs and eliminate the amount of organ waste and inefficiency that, while improving, is not where it could be in our industry."

"Waste, Dr. Finnegan? You talk about the transfer of organs between human beings like we would at our restaurant talking about produce. I don't mean to be disrespectful, but I think describing the transplant process like you are, is, well, abhorrent."

"No need to apologize because you, like many people in the business, are looking at this from the medical perspective, as did I many years ago until I began studying the industry a bit more. There is not a doctor, nurse, or clinician to whom I have explained this that does not look at me at first with the same contempt that I see in your eyes. I think you will begin to see by tackling this problem from a business perspective, we can improve the process from a medical perspective in which the primary and, frankly, the only objective is having more people donate, receive, and survive transplants."

Brooke's silence allowed Dr. Finnegan to continue. "In the transplant business, to increase our yield, if you will, we must have more people giving and getting more organs, and to reduce our spoilage, we have to improve in four basic areas and make major changes in a fifth area." He wrote on the whiteboard in typical illegible doctor scribble:

1. *We need to find more donors before they die. We need to improve the efficiency of matching donors to recipients.*
2. *We need to improve the speed of removing a donated organ from the deceased and transplanting it into the living.*
3. *We need to improve the organ survival rate.*
4. *We need to start thinking about "my body, my choice" when deciding to donate and to whom to donate.*

The first four were the same points Dr. Finnegan covered in detail during the lecture, but Brooke let him continue. What she wanted, though, was to hear about point five, which was the ending slide in the lecture that left the audience shocked.

"You would think our government could help by easing some of the red tape allowing relatives to profit from donating a duplicate organ, such as a kidney, but the only thing the bureaucrats in Washington know how to do is slow things down with red tape. We have had a law on the books since 1984, the National Organ Transplant Act (NOTA), which regulates transplants. That law has been in place for almost 35 years, so we can give up on the government doing anything. In many ways, while the medical side of transplants has improved in leaps and bounds, our puritanical, conservative culture limit advances on the legal side that would keep more of our citizens alive. Do you know Iran, whom we consider barbarians, allows their citizens to sell kidneys? Did you know that 12 people die each day in the United States because they can't get a kidney, which can be a living person donation?"

Brooke did not know the facts about Iran but knew the statistics about kidneys. She stayed quiet, though, and let Dr. Finnegan continue. Almost as if in a trance, he stared at the whiteboard, then as if jolted back to the primary subject at hand, he continued. "It is taboo in our culture to encourage humans to sell their organs, but God forbid we limit their rights to own guns that kill people or make other stupid decisions that endanger their lives and the lives of others. What we can do, though, is take what the laws and government allow us and then perhaps bend the interpretation a bit. The easy improvement The Center has made is point number three, increasing the speed at which the organ is removed from the deceased and placed in the recipient.

As you know, Brooke, many organ transplants occur when a deceased patient dies in, let's say, Little Rock, Arkansas, and has agreed to donate their organs. For example, in instantaneous deaths, like from an accident, speed is critical. The potential donated organs and the patient's other medical records must be uploaded into the UNOS transplant database. Once there, they are matched against potential donors in a 300-mile radius from Little Rock. If we have a perfect match in St. Louis, the organ transplant team gets on a helicopter or private plane, flies down to Little Rock, removes the organ they need, and then flies back to St. Louis to where your team has prepped the patient for surgery. All this takes time.

A few hours to get to Little Rock, an hour to remove the organ, two hours to come back to St. Louis and have the organ in the operating room ready to be placed in your patient. That is five hours if nothing goes wrong. But in the Midwest in the summer, thunderstorms could delay or make air travel incredibly risky."

"The Center is trying to eliminate the process where we fly down and pick out the one or two organs we need, but rather have the body flown here, immediately after death or sometimes when death is hours or days away. This process is difficult, though, because getting a family's permission to have their loved ones whisked away at this critical time is an emotional wreck. We try to archive whole body organ transfers. If we have the whole body here, we can take out all the organs and hopefully have the recipients of the organs only steps away at our Center or the area hospitals, thus eliminating all the travel time."

Brooke interjected, "But, Doctor, you still have travel time because while you may take out the organ of the deceased here at The Center in St. Louis, there is no guarantee the recipients are all here. So you must get the removed organ to the recipient, who may be in a rural area 300 miles away. The government is trying to make an even playing field, so rural patients have enough chance to get an organ as patients near a major medical center or city do."

"True, Brooke, but the core of what we are doing here is eliminating that geographic conflict." Looking at a bowl of fruit on the table, Dr. Finnegan picked up a ripe banana. "Have you ever bought bananas in the store?"

"Yes."

"They are inexpensive, right?" Finnegan asked.

"Sure, I guess," answered Brooke.

"Do you ever wonder how bananas grown in South America can reach St. Louis, thousands of miles away, and sell for around $1.00 for six to seven of them? They're not bruised and usually good to eat two days after you buy them but go bad as quick as four days after you buy them?"

"No, I never wondered about that," Brooke laughed. "But I am wondering why we are talking about bananas?"

"Because the growers pick bananas weeks before they reach the grocery store with these large machines that cut off stalks of bananas hundred, if not thousands at a time, and they are as green as grass. Not ready to eat. Then they ship them in bulk, far in advance of when people need them, so by the time they reach the grocery store, the supply of bananas matches the demand of the consumer wanting the banana. Spoilage is not only minimal, but it is also not the banana grower's problem. At The Center, we want to ensure an increased supply of organs is in the pipeline long before the recipient needs them. We want to control the supply and demand as much as we want to manage spoilage, rejection, and acceptance of an organ."

"That is fascinating, Doctor, but while you tell me how The Center does this, can you hand me that banana? I missed most of my lunch from Dr. Calabrese's questioning. So, I'm a little hungry."

Handing her the banana and grabbing a Power Bar for himself, he continued, "As I said, there is little The Center can impact if death occurs instantly and not within our building. So, we focus on the donor and recipient well before death occurs."

"And how do you do that?"

"We market to them, just like any business selling a product. Part of what you saw in the GUTS room is our marketing and outreach center to donors and recipients. The UNOS national database manages those who have agreed to donate organs to those who need organs. We use our GUTS technology to increase potential supply by finding people who may be terminal but have not agreed to be organ donors or believe they have the right to choose when to die and, when they do, the right to choose who gets their organ. We reached out to them with our presentation on The Center, which is why the Ortel and Johnson families came to our Center. I believe organ donation is constrained because some potential donors, as they do with many things in their life, want a plan, how they die, and where their organs go. Organ donations do not have to involve the loss of a loved one and no knowledge of where the organs are going. I believe organs, the donor's family, and the recipient and their family fare much better if they know each other before the transplant.

We try to minimize the anguish and sorrow for the donor family and the guilt and questions the recipient's family has. Doing so creates a bond between families that help organs prosper. Most of the time, we work within the guidelines outlined by the Health and Human Services, Organ Procurement and Transplant Network (OPTN). As we grow our pipeline of patients who want choice, we also are incorporating our guidelines that will begin to challenge conventional thinking."

"Doctor, I know you talked about choice in your seminar, but really, how viable is that concept, either legally or morally?" Brooke asked.

"Yes, I will get to that and how you may be part of that. But let me ask you, have you seen the guilt and questions from the recipient and the family in your job? Who is donating my organ? How did the person die? What were their lifestyle choices?"

"You're right. In almost all cases, beyond fear of the actual operation, the recipient fears the organ's health and has questions and guilt about the person who donated," Brooke said. "As grateful as they should be to get the gift of life, I am shocked how everyday embedded prejudice and judgment come into play by the patient and even more so by family members. I have had many patients ask me if they must "take" an organ from someone of a different race, religion, gender, and even if you can believe it, political party."

"Brooke, we plan to eliminate all that by advocating for the donor's right to choose where their organs go. Take the Johnson and Ortel families. Sam Johnson has advanced stages of dementia. So, his family knows he will die soon, and they have graciously agreed to donate his organs but on their terms. Chuck Ortel knows he needs the heart to survive. They have both agreed to become part of The Center's vision because they choose to become intertwined in life and death. As they get to know each other, they feel more comfortable knowing that his heart is going to a good man. Now because we follow the rules, we know Sam Johnson is not in the UNOS database, so we are not plucking him off that list and putting him on our list. We are giving Sam a choice, and he chose our process. Mr. Ortel has also chosen our approach. He could get his care from a hospital and let the UNOS database choose whose organs he may or may not get, but he does not want to take that chance. He wants more control, and he wants to know his donor. Control is precisely what The Center gives him: control over his body and his choice.

"But I only saw Mr. Ortel's family, and Mr. Johnson said he is donating several organs. What about those families?"

"Good question, Brooke. If other families do not agree to come to The Center in advance to meet Mr. Johnson, then when he passes, Mr. Johnson's organs are contributed to the national database, and those go to the best match from UNOS. We will not waste any of Mr. Johnson's other organs as we will remove them. Hopefully, because he is here in The Center, we will have a recipient for his organs just minutes away, either in The Center or at a hospital. Like bananas Brooke, the key is to have lots of donors before they are needed. We believe the recipients will learn what we are trying to do here and make every effort to stay at The Center and meet their donors. We will also try and use group meeting software like ZOOM to have the families meet, but we prefer they come to The Center.

"Is that because the success rate is better?" Brooke asked.

"That, and we make more money from insurance if both the donor and recipient stay at The Center. We want control of the entire operation, so to speak, for all the organs, the donors, and recipients. Remember, Brooke, it is a business after all. Supply, demand, elimination of spoilage, and customer satisfaction. Any questions so far, Brooke?"

"About a hundred, but one big one is point five on your board. I get what you are trying to do on the first four points, but the fifth one, as you described, seems like it would not withstand legal and moral challenges," Brooke said.

"What's more immoral, Brooke? Have people die because there are not enough organs? Or not giving people a choice when or how they die, or to whom to give their organs? I think how our society views transplants, and life and death decisions are more immoral than anything I have outlined. I know my ideas make medical people, investors, politicians, and religious zealots squirm, and I know I will be sued by every court in the land, but this is my vision. It will either revolutionize this industry and make me rich, a pariah, or worse, have me end up in prison."

Brooke wanted to ask Dr. Finnegan many more questions, especially about the legality of his concept. Before she could, though, he took a phone call and said to Brooke that he had to run as one of the donors had passed away, and he needed to prep for the operation.

"Not Mr. Johnson, I hope," she said.

Dr. Finnegan did not answer but said, "Brooke, let me walk you to the elevator, and if you can see yourself out, that would be great. The operating room awaits. Maybe you can come by another day and see that aspect of The Center."

As they waited for the elevator doors to open, Dr. Finnegan looked at Brooke and said, "Point five is all about choices. The ones we make in life, the ones we make before death, but society and laws don't allow it. The Transplant Center is all about choosing both life and death, and I plan to put the control back where it belongs: outside of the government and back to the people whose life depends on it."

Before she could ask Dr. Finnegan any more questions, the elevator doors opened. As Dr. Finnegan walked away, he turned back to Brooke, who had now gotten into the elevator, and said, "Brooke, point five is an important discussion for another day that I hope we get to share soon."

The door closed, and she pushed L for the lobby. Her head was spinning from what she had just heard. She once read somewhere geniuses were madmen with better clothes. After listening to Dr. Finnegan, she knew he was a genius. She was not sure just yet if he also wasn't a madman.

CHAPTER 22

Frank and Sue had dinner at their home and invited Vinnie, who was shocked at how difficult it was for Frank to breathe. Further shocking was the number of portable oxygen cylinders that now filled almost every open area on the first floor of their home. This visit was the first chance Vinnie had to visit Frank since his diagnosis, and he was not ready for the encounter. Vinnie had never been comfortable around illness or sick people, but he tried to hide his uneasiness around Frank and Sue.

During one of their many gatherings, their dining room table was usually filled with ample food and ever-growing family and friends. Things were smaller nowadays due to Frank's illness. Vinnie was last here on Christmas Eve when Sue had prepared a traditional Italian dinner called Night of the Seven Fishes.

Tonight's meal, although small, still consisted of several classic Italian dishes. Plates of gnocchi. Bowls of sausages and meatballs. Salad. And, of course, a plethora of trays filled with Sue's famous pastries, including Angel Wings: a sweet, deep-fried pastry made of dough, twisted into thin ribbons, and finally sprinkled with powdered sugar and honey. Those were Vinnie's favorites since he and Sue were children, watching their mother and grandmother prepare comparable feasts of Italian delicacies.

Even with the warmth of full bellies, tonight's dinner was more somber. Vinnie saw Frank's difficulty moving from the couch to the table. As if that wasn't enough heartache, Frank had to stop between nearly every sip of liquid and every bite of food to breathe. Many times, that was made worse by frequent and extended violent coughing fits.

The phrase *"coughing up a lung"* came to Vinnie's mind while Frank gained some stability in his breathing and the coughing stopped. While Vinnie was uncomfortable and at a loss for words, an unusual state of mind for him, Frank seemed outwardly unfazed by his condition. He continued the conversation between coughing spasms, jumping from subject to subject, asking first how Vinnie, his kids, and grandkids were, and asking about Ellen. Despite the divorce from Vinnie, Ellen was still close to Frank and Sue.

Vinnie did not know whether to give short answers or long; both intended to manage how much Frank would need to talk in response. Vinnie asked Frank about his work, and surprisingly, Frank was still working from home at his job as a lead technical program manager for Master-Card. They talked about kids, some gossip about their other siblings and relatives, some sports, and a little politics. The latter two subjects were ones in which Frank had little interest. Soon the conversation seemed natural, but during it, Vinnie looked at Frank and wondered: *how the hell could he go on? How can Frank still be cheerful? Isn't he afraid of the future?* But that was Frank and Sue: always positive.

After a while and to do less talking, Frank brought out the cards and wine. They played a few hands of gin rummy while Vinnie and Sue had some of Frank's homemade wine. With Vinnie a bit more relaxed because of the wine, he probed a little more on how Frank was feeling and how he and Sue were coping. In most conversations, Vinnie was usually unfiltered and got quickly to the point, even asking uncomfortable or blunt personal questions. Tonight though, with Frank and Sue, he trod a little lighter.

"So Frank, what happens next?" Vinnie asked.

"Well, I still need to get in better shape and lose another 15 pounds before I am eligible to get a transplant," Frank said, pausing to breathe. "It has been hard to have the energy to do that. I started on two oxygen concentrators, and they were supplying about 6-8 liters per minute (LPM) of oxygen, but now I need to use both the concentrators and the tanks since I am going through 15-20 LPMs. I am going through so much of these it is difficult for our local supplier to fulfill." Frank paused again and then continued, "My needs are increasing just to breathe. So, next week I am going back to Barnes to talk to them about a better solution."

Vinnie thought it took Frank two minutes to tell him 30 seconds' worth of information. All Vinnie could ask was: "Is all of this covered by insurance?" Vinnie knew that over the last few years, Frank had been doing mostly contract work and was unsure if he had insurance or if Sue had coverage in her job as a teacher's aide.

Frank answered, "Oh, you did not hear, I guess. I got picked up by Citicorp as a full-time employee after my latest contract assignment with them, so we have full insurance now."

That was probably the best news Vinnie had heard since he got here. He was very concerned about insurance and the mounting costs Frank and Sue were absorbing.

"What about the transplant time frame? Are you on a donor list yet?" Vinnie asked.

"No, not yet, and they won't put me on the list until I cross the threshold of dire sickness and good health. Pretty screwed up, huh?" said Frank.

"Well, I would have used the word pretty fucked-up, but then again, I am not as polite as you," Vinnie laughed.

Sue and Frank nodded in agreement, but Frank soon went from laughing to violently coughing. When he caught his breath, Frank told Vinnie that as bad as he was, he had seen people worse than him at the transplant rehab center at Barnes. People he saw a month ago, he guessed, were no longer alive today if they had not gotten a transplant.

That's fucked-up, Vinnie thought to himself, this time silently. That thought sobered Vinnie up a bit which was a good thing as the evening was getting late, and Vinnie still had an hour's drive back home to St. Louis. He began to prepare to leave but not before Sue, not surprising-ly, pulled out a take-home tray of pastries, including his favorite Angel Wings. Knowing Vinnie was coming over, she had made a small batch, which was no easy task. Angel Wings are very complicated and time-consuming.

Saying goodbyes with a hug for Sue but keeping some distance from Frank, Vinnie told them to call him if there was anything he could do. They promised they would.

As Vinnie got in his truck and looked down at the plate of Angel Wings, he thought, *that is what Frank needs, Angel Wings to guide him to good health.* Not being very religious, Vinnie thought it hypocritical to ask God for favors, and besides, he was sure that was not how it worked. Vinnie silently prayed anyway, asking the big guy upstairs to look over Frank. He then reached down, took an Angel Wing, dripping with honey and powdered sugar, and as if to offer it up as a communion host during mass, Vinnie lifted it, put it in his mouth, and then drove off.

CHAPTER 23

D etective Simon seemed to be at a dead end with all her active cases. While she was concerned about solving them, she was not concerned about being idle for long because killing never took more than a 36–72-hour breather in St. Louis. Most of her murder investigations involved drug dealers or drug usage that had gone bad. Her second most frequent murder motive was domestic violence between husbands and wives. Or violence from an estranged or hidden lover wanting to come out behind the shadows. Lastly, carjacking's gone wrong, either for the victim or the carjacker. Since carjacking has been on the rise, many more carjackers found themselves on the receiving end of a gun as more and more citizens were carrying a weapon in their car, either legally or illegally. What bothered Detective Simon most about carjackings was that the perpetrators were becoming younger, in many cases 13-17 years old. The motive was usually a gang initiation as they never took the car for more than a quick ride before dumping it.

Their course curriculum in this level of crime education was to prove they could stick a gun in someone's face and take the car. Like getting extra credit points on a final exam, if for some reason the car owner was killed in the process, they may earn a higher score in the eyes of the gangs. Maybe they rifled through the glove box and trunk to see if anything was worth stealing, but they never cashed in by taking the car to a chop shop or selling it as a stolen vehicle.

The other troubling aspect of carjacking was the randomness of the victim. Most carjackings took place in the neighborhoods where criminals lived, in the wee hours of the morning, when decent citizens should be home sleeping. In about 50% of carjackings, the crimes occurred between 10:30 p.m.-3:00 a.m., usually on a busy thoroughfare running through a downtown bar district or neighborhood gathering spot. When people assembled to have a good time, people congregated to make trouble. It was human nature.

The other 50% of carjackings occurred where you would least expect it and to whom you would least expect it. The tapping of a bumper at a busy intersection in broad daylight, a woman, innocently shopping at a grocery or department store with her kids in tow. The mall parking lots were very popular and accessible. Large amounts of cars, low visibility, and the victim usually burdened by the fumbling shopping bags while putting them in their vehicles, making them vulnerable. The other increasingly popular carjacking venue was sporting events, and, on this evening, it was a sporting event where Detective Simon headed.

A shooting occurred in a parking lot two blocks south of Busch Stadium on 7th and Cerre Street, between two popular bars, Paddy O's and Kilroy's. This lot was just one of the dozens filled by fans attending tonight's Cardinal game.

Usually, the only issues before or after a Cardinals' game were public drunkenness, which resulted in an occasional fight between opposing teams' fans. But that was rare as baseball fans were polite, especially Cardinals fans, and because baseball seasons had so many games, it was rare to rile up fans unless that one loss was a do-or-die moment.

Even when the Chicago Cubs were in town, the Cardinals' oldest and fiercest rival, the fan interaction mainly was good-natured ribbing. If a fight happened to break out between the teams' fans, friends of the fighters typically stepped into breakup drunken banter before it turned into sloppy fist fights.

Violent crime was even less of a problem, not because of the gentile nature of baseball fans but more so the incredible police presence on every corner within a 1-mile radius of the stadium. The Cardinals franchise and the stadium were the crown jewels of St. Louis. When it would have been so easy to move to the suburbs, their presence downtown was more valuable, both in prestige and economics, than the Gateway Arch or all the downtown restaurants. If downtown was to continue to have a pulse, it was in the veins of the 40,000 fans each night that came to see a game. Because of this, there were more cops than t-shirts and peanut vendors on game night. That's not to say that violent crime did not happen, but usually, it was an outlier, happening beyond the glare of the stadium lights or much later in the evening, long after the game was over, when most fans had headed home.

Detective Simon wondered about this shooting as the call came in at 8:30 p.m. while the game started at 7:10 p.m., was not over. The location was so close to the stadium that you could hear the crowd roar over the fireworks going off to celebrate a Cardinals' homerun. Plus, the area was between two very popular bars. Maybe a lover's quarrel? Maybe a scuffle between scalpers and their customers over fake tickets? She wasn't sure about the motive but did not have a good feeling about this one as she pulled onto 7th street and into the parking lot where the shooting occurred. The significant presence of what seemed to be all 200 cops that patrolled Busch stadium plus child welfare services set off an alarm. Was a child also involved?

As she left her car and elbowed her way between the medical and police presence, she did hear the wail of a child screaming inconsolably. Soon she saw the little boy, around 5 or 6 years old, with light blonde hair, shaking, crying, screaming, and trying to be consoled by a child welfare officer. Leaning into the ear of the officer, Simon whispered, "Get him out of here. He should not see this."

The officer turned around with a tear in her eye. "Unfortunately, it is too late for that," and as she did, she pointed subtly to her left where, although hidden for the time being from Simon's and the child's view, was the body of the victim. As the police officers parted a bit and Simon eased through, she first saw the blue tarp covering the victim, and as she walked around to turn down the portion covering the victim's head, she looked back to where the child was to make sure he had been taken away. He had, and she then removed the tarp to look at the victim's face, or what was left of it, as it had been torn apart by a bullet fired at very close range.

Simon sighed and took a deep breath. Simon was a hardened homicide detective. She had seen hundreds of scenes like this, but she was also human and needed a moment to compose herself. She knew some aspects of a crime scene triggered the sickening feeling she had now. Whenever a child was in any way involved, it got to her. Whenever she saw a victim that was indeed an innocent bystander, minding their own business, it got to her. Whenever she saw herself in the victim's surroundings, that got to her, too. Hell, she had parked in this lot many times taking her kids and grandkids to a Cardinals' game, and from the look of the victim and a guess at his age, it seemed the child was his grandson. *"Damn it,"* Simon said to herself, *"You can't even be safe taking your grandchild to a fucking ball game."*

Pausing just a little longer before she covered the victim's head, she turned to the crowd of cops, composed herself and without showing any of the emotion that she felt 30 seconds ago, simply asked, "So, what do we have?"

Looking into the eyes of her fellow cops, she could tell a few shared the emotions she was having, but there was something more in their eyes. It was vengeance and hatred. These emotions usually came out at an after-hours bar hangout filled with cops, but this was more visceral. Most of the beat cops working the stadium shift got to do so because it was a cushy gig earned by seniority, and most of the cops who had seniority were older and whiter and more akin to the victim lying at their feet.

In the summer heat, emotions always ran high between cops and the public. It seemed every summer there was protest and tension over police brutality, whether the police action occurred in St. Louis directly or St. Louis, like most major cities, erupted in protest from a national story happening elsewhere. She sensed that the cops had already labeled the perpetrator and were ready to hand out some street justice.

"Who was first on the scene here?" Simon asked; now, all business.

"I was, Detective," offered a patrol officer named McGarrity. Revenge, hatred, anger. Simon could see it in McGarrity's 60-year-old eyes. She knew McGarrity saw himself as the victim. Simon would win a wager that McGarrity had grandkids and took them to ball games.

"Ok, McGarrity, give me your take on what went down."

"Well, we think the victim, named William Thomson, left the ball game early, as it was only about the 5th inning, and we think the shooting occurred around 8:15. I guess that he had his hands full with his grandson, as well as some souvenirs and a soft-sided cooler, which we found in the back seat of the car." McGarrity paused to take a deep breath. Simon obliged as she sensed this was difficult for him as if he had walked in the victim's footprints many times.

"Both the driver's and driver's side passenger doors were open. The car keys were on the front seat of the driver's side. The grandson was in the car seat, unbuckled though when we arrived. The victim, we believe, put his grandson into the car seat, and while his back was turned to the parking lot, the son of a bitch shot him in the back of the head. We have large blood splatters on the top of the car and inside the car, primarily in the rear seats and on his grandson in the car seat."

Simon gave McGarrity a few more seconds to compose himself as she sensed he was about to burst into anger or tears, and she knew he would be thankful that his emotions were not in full view of his fellow officers. Still, Simon knew plenty of them were feeling the same way.

"Do you think the victim tried to resist, fight back in any way?" Simon probed.

"Not sure. There are shoe patterns on the crushed stone in the parking lot where maybe a brief scuffle occurred. It's hard to tell whose they are, though, or if they were made by Mr. Thomson scuffling his feet while trying to wrangle his grandson in the seat. Anyone who has ever tried to put a child in a car seat knows how that wrestling match can happen from time to time," McGarrity said with experience in his voice.

"Do you think straight robbery or carjacking?" Simon asked McGarrity, knowing it did not matter.

And as if reading Simon's mind, McGarrity said, "Does it matter? A guy is taking his grandkid to the game." McGarrity spoke in halting, hindered breaths. "Probably having the time of their lives. Kid needs to get home early or is tired or bored of the game," his voice quivering, "had his fill of cotton candy and hot dogs. Walking to his car, probably reminiscing about the memory they will have for a lifetime, then boom, some asshole, some fucking loser, decides now is the time to gain some street cred. Let's rob this old guy. Let's take his car. FUCK!" McGarrity yelled at the top of his lungs and broke down simultaneously.

"Fuck indeed, McGarrity," Simon said, finishing McGarrity's thoughts. "Punk plans to rob or jack the guy, but maybe seeing Thomson has a child with him, maybe that scares him off the carjacking, so after the scuffle, he grabs his wallet and runs off. I get the robbery, but only true evil shoots a person in cold blood in front of a child." The remaining patrol officers nod their heads in agreement as they console McGarrity and each other.

As the coroner lifted Mr. Thomson's body into the back of their vehicle, the sound of fireworks from the stadium erupted, indicating a Cardinal win. Simon thought, *What a fucking mess of a world. Forty thousand fans go home happy tonight, but one family's life is shattered. True evil is lurking on the streets tonight.*

Simon asked the patrol officers if there were any witnesses. The officers didn't look up, only down at the pavement, shaking their heads. Simon looked out past Thomson's car east into the parking lot, now filled with revelers from the game about to get in their cars and head home. They were curious as to why there were so many police here, but none stopped to ask why as if they already knew it wouldn't be good news. Simon then walked a few steps out to 7th street and looked north towards the stadium and then south towards the historic Soulard district. She was not sure what she was looking for or at, but her gaze went past the stream of cars headed towards Interstates 44 and 55 and onto the corner of the Eat-Rite Diner, a greasy spoon loved by drunks and panhandlers from midnight till dawn.

On the corner stood two young men. No shirts covered their muscular yet thin chests and glistening brown skin. Pants pulled down past their navels, revealing their underwear: the fashion statement of the inner-city youth. She caught their eye, and they returned the stare with a mixture of menace and indifference. Based on the movement of their mouths, Simon could tell they were saying, "Fuck you" back to her, shooting a finger in the air and taking off south laughing. Simon did not give chase. With all the congestion, they couldn't get far anyway, and there was no reason to believe they were part of the shooting. Their hatred of the police was every day. Before they returned to the neighborhood they came from, they stopped and talked briefly to a driver in a white car pulled to the side of 7th street, maybe 100 feet away from the westbound Interstate 44/55 entrance. She was too far away to see the car brand or license plate. It stopped for a few seconds as the men got in, then raced west on the interstate.

CHAPTER 24

Brooke could not get her mind off what she saw and heard at the Transplant Center the previous day. What confused her was that it seemed to make sense but contradicted most of everything she knew about the transplant process. The current process had flaws, all expertly pointed out by Dr. Finnegan and Dr. Calabrese, but what bothered her was how they took a medical miracle and packaged it as a business algorithm. She had spent many nights sitting with her patients and families, sharing their joy of getting a transplant and the sorrow when they were passed over.

Whenever Brooke was troubled, as she was now, she turned to her best source of advice, her mom and dad, discussing whatever was on her mind over a cup of coffee and apple pie at her family's restaurant.

Pulling into the parking lot, which unfortunately was emptier than it should be for the lunch hour, Brooke entered through the back kitchen door, greeted some of the long-term employees that they could keep on, and immediately headed to the large coffee urn. She poured herself a cup of coffee and then grabbed a slice of apple pie from the pastry refrigerator. And because she was feeling a little down, she scooped a large dollop of whipped cream on top of the pie.

Walking toward the employee break room, she saw her father prepping some of the lunch orders. Holding up her cup of coffee and pie, she motioned to him to meet her there. He nodded instinctively as coffee and pie were their universal code language for "let's talk."

Even with the slightly empty parking lot, Brooke's mom and dad were busy serving the lunch crowd and handling takeout orders. With everyone working, the breakroom was completely open. Her dad usually patrolled the kitchen, and her mom was the front-of-the-house greeter and server if needed. Brooke settled in with her coffee and pie, knowing not to wait on her parents as they could be tied up for a few minutes or an hour, depending on the busyness of the restaurant. She and her sisters had spent many hours in the break room, doing homework after school, treating friends to some food, or, as she was doing now, talking to her parents about a problem. She and her parents liked using the break room instead of a restaurant table because invariably, they would be interrupted by friends and regulars stopping by to say hi, compliment them on the food and service, or in very rare cases, complain about something. MacIntoshes was not only a family restaurant but also a community tradition and meeting place, and the break room offered a bit more privacy for family discussions.

After 10 minutes, long enough for Brooke to finish her pie and grab a second cup of coffee, her father came in and, after a quick squeeze and hug of his little Brookie, as he liked to call her, settled in a chair.

"So Brookie, apple pie, with whipped cream. It must be a heck of a problem you have resting on your beautiful shoulders. But if it's man trouble, let me get your mother," he said, which was his standard response on anything relationship-oriented.

"No, dad, not man problems, or women problems, in case you are wondering," she said. "More of an ethical problem."

"I think ethics are also your mom's domain," he laughed. "I handle the simple stuff, solved quickly."

"Well, unfortunately for you, I think you are the guy for this problem, and as I said, I am not sure it is a problem versus a question or two. Maybe you should get a piece of pie and settle in."

Her dad, patting his belly, indicating more pie was not in the cards, sat silently and let Brooke continue.

"Do you think it is right to profit on the misfortune of others?"

Again, silence from her father as he waited for Brooke to unwind her thoughts.

Knowing she needed to expand a bit more to get her father to budge off his silent perch, she went on as he believed the best way to get someone to talk was to listen.

"I visited a company called Arch City Transplant Center and met with two brilliant or possibly insane doctors who gave me a tour of the facility. I don't know; maybe they were even interviewing me for a job. Have you heard of them?"

"Honey, unless it is something I can cook, eat or serve, you know I am not very knowledgeable about things outside my restaurant kingdom here. So no, I have not heard of them."

Brooke wasn't surprised that her dad had not heard of them as he usually thought 24/7 about the restaurant, especially during the pandemic, but he sold himself short on his level of knowledge. Her dad was an encyclopedia and could absorb large amounts of information by listening and consuming news snippets. She also knew that as soon as she walked out of the restaurant, he would be googling Arch City Transplant, so the next time they talked, he would be ready with all sorts of advice, wanted or unwanted by her.

"So, what's the deal with them. Are you thinking of making a job change?"

"No. Maybe. I am not sure the Doctors were even interviewing me. Maybe they were providing me with information as a professional courtesy. Since, in a way, I am a peer of theirs because of my job at the hospital. I just got a weird vibe that they were feeling me out about their operation, like testing me to see if I objected to their approach or could be an ally of theirs."

Brooke then went on and explained Arch City in layman's terms and covered her time there in about five minutes due to her dad's dwindling patience as he constantly looked out at the kitchen, ensuring his staff had the orders handled.

"Well, Brooke, I am not sure about all the technical stuff or the personalities of the two doctors. But in response to your initial question, while I don't think it is right to profit from the misfortunate of others, I do not think that is what they are doing at Arch City. It seems like they are trying to fix a process that might be broken, and if they can make money from it, so be it. You always tell me about the pain and misfortune your transplant patients and their families suffer. So, maybe Arch City's approach lessens that pain. But what do I know? I am just a burger flipper at a restaurant."

"Well, Dad, you may be the smartest and most insightful burger flipper I know, and not all burger flippers can understand and summarize complex subjects into a sound piece of advice. So, thank you."

"You are always welcome, Brookie, but I am not sure of the motives of that Finnegan guy. He seems shifty to me. Keep an eye on him."

Leaving that comment lay and knowing her time with her dad was over, she began to rise from her chair but heard her phone ping, indicating an inbound text. She glanced at it quickly, seeing it was from Dr. Ellen James- Calabrese. It read: "RU free to meet for lunch over the next couple of days? I wanted to follow up on our meeting. LMK. Thanks."

Brooke tossed her phone back into her purse, not responding to the text. She hugged her dad and then went to the hostess stand to say hi to her mom.

CHAPTER 25

Several weeks after Vinnie visited with Sue and Frank, he got a text from Frank asking if he could give him a lift to his next rehab session at the hospital. Not having a full schedule or any schedule since he retired, Vinnie agreed and, on Wednesday, took the hour drive to Frank's house to pick him up.

It had been only two weeks since he last saw Frank, but it seemed like two years ago based on how frail Frank now looked. Vinnie was shocked at the deterioration of Frank's health in such a short period. When he parked in the driveway of Frank and Sue's house, Sue came out and asked him to pull into the garage, so it would be easier for Frank to get into the truck.

Vinnie obliged, thinking, *What difference do 25 feet make from being in the driveway or the garage?* As soon as he entered the house, he knew why it made a difference.

When he had visited two weeks prior, Frank was moving slowly; being tethered to portable oxygen tanks would do that, but now his movements were prolonged and labored. While still greeting Vinnie with his ever-present smile, Vinnie wondered if Frank's days would soon end.

With Sue's aid, Vinnie helped Frank into the front seat of his truck while Sue moved his oxygen tanks to the back seat and carefully uncoiled the air tubes connecting the tanks to Frank. Once secure and settled in,

Sue kissed Frank goodbye, and he and Vinnie began their drive back towards St. Louis to Barnes Hospital.

As bad as Frank looked physically, his spirits and his conversation were lively as ever. He and Vinnie chatted on the way to the hospital on various subjects as if they were two guys going to play golf. Vinnie kept the conversation light, and while he wanted to understand what Frank was thinking or feeling about his health and future, now was not the time. And besides, Frank was the most positive person Vinnie knew, and while not saying it, Frank probably believed everything would work out fine. After 30 minutes, they pulled into the drop-off area of the rehab center, where a rehab coordinator met them and assisted Frank and his tanks out of the car. Even though there were wheelchairs available, Frank and the coordinator walked into the rehab center.

As he pulled away, Vinnie noticed several people, who looked like patients, standing on the sidewalk smoking cigarettes. While not sure they were patients, Vinnie still shook his head, wondering how people, whoever they were, could smoke outside a rehab center where others, perhaps their relatives or friends, went to rehab to get healthy enough to get a transplant. While humanity always amazed Vinnie with acts of kindness and generosity, individuals disgusted Vinnie with their stupidity.

After parking his truck in the garage, Vinnie returned to the rehab lobby. To his surprise, Frank was still in the waiting area.

"They are not ready for me yet," Frank said to Vinnie as Vinnie sat down next to him.

Since they had a few minutes, Vinnie felt comfortable asking Frank a little more about what happens during rehab and the transplant process.

"What do you do in there?" Vinnie asked, pointing to the door that indicated it was for patients and staff only.

"Well, it's just like a small fitness center for very sick people. They put me on a treadmill monitoring me with a pulse oximeter that measures oxygen concentration levels. It needs to stay 90% or above, and I must walk half a mile in 30 minutes with an oxygen flow of 20 liters."

Knowing it usually takes about 20 minutes to walk a mile at an effortless pace, Vinnie did the math in his head and thought that Frank would be barely moving at that pace. Wondering how to avoid saying something stupid like *well, that sounds easy enough*; he just asked, "Are you up to the levels you need to be to get the transplant?"

Frank replied, "I'm not there yet, but if I can get up to the level needed and sustain it, I can be eligible for a transplant."

Frank was then called into the rehab center, and as he shuffled off, Vinnie yelled out, "Hey, don't push yourself just to impress the ladies." As soon as the words left his mouth, Vinnie thought, *that was stupid."* The glum stares from others waiting to go into rehab confirmed that.

Forty-five minutes later, Frank emerged and said, "All done, let's get out of here." Vinnie left to get his truck and was back at the pickup area a few minutes later. After getting Frank and his oxygen tanks secure and settled, they headed off. Since it was near lunchtime, Frank said, "I am hungry. Do you want to get lunch before heading home? My treat."

Vinnie could always eat, so they drove into the Central West End, a trendy shopping and entertainment area lined with stately old trees on private streets with early 20th-century era mansions – streets only the richest had access. They wanted to find a restaurant with outdoor seating to be safer for Frank. Vinnie was looking forward to having lunch, one because he was hungry, and two because he had many more questions for Frank. Some were very personal, but he felt it was an excellent time to ask. Settling in at one of the outside tables at Mission Taco, Vinnie, uncharacteristically for him, asked Frank if he minded answering a few more questions.

Frank, knowing Vinnie was never shy about asking questions, nodded in acknowledgment as if saying, "fire away."

"I guess the first thing I wonder about is the people at rehab. Are they all there getting conditioned for lung transplants? Is this who you are competing with to get a lung?"

"Well," Frank said, pulling his mask down to eat a chip, "I am not sure who is all there. Some are awaiting lung transplants. I see them and talk to them regularly, while others already may have had a transplant or are rehabbing for something else."

"But do you ever feel that the guy or woman you are talking to might get lungs instead of you?"

"No, not really. I want everyone to get lungs or whatever they need. If they are before me, it's because they are sicker than I am, or they are a better match. I worry that the very sick ones I know may only be weeks away from dying without a transplant. I don't feel I am sick enough to go to the head of the line, but it does not work like that anyway," Frank continued.

Vinnie thought about Frank's compassion for others as Frank would put someone else's needs ahead of his own.

"Do you see the same people all the time at rehab? Do you know when someone gets tapped on the shoulder, so to speak, that it's their turn?" Vinnie asked rapidly.

Frank replied, "Well, I know some people because we may be on the same rehab schedule, but I think we all know that we will be in rehab for only a short period, and the different outcomes are stark. Either someone quits going to rehab because they got a lung, or they didn't, and they are no longer here."

Vinnie did not have to ask about the people who didn't get a lung or a set of lungs. He knew the answer.

Frank was able to fill in the blanks of what Vinnie was thinking. "What gets me is the people I meet who work so hard to get in better shape to accept a transplant, but they never get one because they don't find a match. They just run out of time, or someone is a better match, and they get passed up," Frank added.

Vinnie wished Frank had not brought up this topic because it was something that Vinnie always had in his mind, partly because if Frank had any luck in life, it seemed bad luck.

"So, what do you need for a match?" Vinnie hesitantly asked.

"Well, the key things for a lung transplant are blood type match as well as body type match," Frank explained.

"What do you mean body type? Like from another guy your age? Does he have to be a white guy?" Vinnie peppered Frank with questions before he had time to answer.

"No, not a white guy, or even a guy. They do not have to be my age either. The lung has to just fit. For example, look at that big guy over there." Frank pointed to another person who had just walked in. "That guy must be six foot five, so his lungs are big, probably bigger than mine. He would not be a good match, or I don't think he would."

Vinnie looked over at the person, looked back at Frank, and nodded in understanding. "Well, if that's the case, you begin to limit the number of people whose lungs may be available to you, right?"

"Yes, but because of that and my lung disease has no cure, nor any interest in slowing down its attack on my body, I agreed to take any person's lung that matches my blood type and body type."

"When you say any person, what do you mean?"

"I mean anybody. A man, a woman, a drug addict, an alcoholic, a criminal. Black, White, Asian, Arab, Hispanic. Atheist, Christian, Muslim. Anybody," Frank said with a high degree of urgency in his voice. The urgency was a first for Vinnie. He had not heard that from Frank in past conversations.

Vinnie just nodded, thinking and doing what he always did in tense situations, reverted to sarcastic humor. "Even a Trump supporter?"

"Yes, Vinnie, even a Trump supporter." Frank laughed loudly until his laughter became a violent coughing fit, and Vinnie wished Frank was not such a smart ass at times like this.

Seeing how the coughing fit had made other diners around them shift uneasily in their seats and sensing how the long day was beginning to take its toll on Frank, Vinnie grabbed the check before Frank could. He threw down $40 to cover the bill and tip, and they walked slowly back to Vinnie's truck.

The ride back to Frank's house was quiet, with Frank dozing a bit and Vinnie lost in his thoughts. In his mind, Vinnie went over two things. The first is: *this is so fucked up.* The second is: *how much longer Frank has before his time runs out.* When they arrived at Frank and Sue's house, Vinnie pulled into the garage again. Vinnie helped Frank back inside and then headed back to his own home. On the way, he kept repeating the same two thoughts repeatedly, but this time, a third thought popped into his head. *How the hell did I get so lucky to avoid being this sick?*

CHAPTER 26

Dr. Ellen James-Calabrese and Brooke agreed to meet for a late lunch on Friday at Sunset Country Club before Ellen met with Alex Finnegan and some investors later that afternoon at the club. Alex was taking the investors golfing and afterward treating them to cocktails to loosen their wallets up and then dinner if they weren't loose enough to add a few more zeros to their investment. Ellen would join them for cocktails and possibly dinner, depending upon how drunk they were from a day on the course. No matter what status she achieved in life, now as the Chief Medical Officer of the Transplant Center or as a well-established surgeon, when the booze flowed, it seemed the inappropriate comments from men to her only increased. Ellen knew that no matter how wealthy and successful these men were, they acted the same as any lout at the corner bar. These guys were just better-dressed letches and craftier at how they hurled their sexual innuendos to her or any woman.

Ellen thought a woman like Brooke, young and beautiful, probably had to deal with this sort of bullshit more often than she did, but she also sensed that Brooke, smart as she was, could handle herself well. It was one of the reasons she was so drawn to Brooke when they first met on the tour of the Transplant Center. Brooke had strong, silent confidence, and she reminded Ellen of herself when she was younger. Not that Ellen lacked confidence, but the confidence of a 30-year-old woman comes from a different source than the confidence of a 58-year-old woman.

With the afternoon summer heat blazing, Ellen quickly chose the comfort of a table in the air-conditioned Club Room, which still came with a beautiful view despite being inside. Besides, the outside area was usually filled with men finishing golf, grabbing lunch, and sharing revelry, especially those wanting to get their weekend started on a Friday afternoon. Ellen got to the club room about 10 minutes early, as it was always more comfortable for a guest if the member was there before to greet them, and today's lunch was all about making Brooke more comfortable with Ellen. Brooke entered the dining room promptly at 2:00, escorted by Scott, the lead server in the afternoon. She dressed in a beautiful, casual blue pastel sundress and dressy sandals complemented by a summer tan.

Taking Brooke directly to the table, surrounded by the stares of several suddenly attentive male diners, Scott pulled out a chair for Brooke and, as he had done a thousand times, said, "Dr. Calabrese, your guest has arrived. May I start your weekend off early by offering you a glass of wine on this beautiful Friday afternoon?"

"Well, that sounds good for me because I am not going back to work," Ellen replied, "but Brooke, is it the weekend yet for you?"

"I have been at work since 6:00 a.m. and don't need to return. So yes, I think the weekend starts now. Anything you suggest, Dr. Calabrese, is fine with me."

"I suggest you stop calling me Dr. Calabrese. Then I suggest the Rombauer Chardonnay. Does that sound good, Brooke, on both suggestions?"

"Ok, Doctor, I mean, Ellen. Sorry, you have me out of my natural element. This may take a while getting used to," Brooke said with a smile, indicating she was beginning to relax around Ellen.

Pleased that she had gotten Brooke to relax, Ellen probed, "So, what is your natural element, Brooke? What does a young woman like yourself do for fun in old boring St. Louis?"

"Well, not that I do it for fun, but I work a lot. Love it. I would work seven days a week if it were not so intense. But for fun, I run a lot and hike in the area parks. Love to swim, kayak, anything involving the water or nature." She looked over the golf course and added, "I don't play golf, but this is beautiful."

"How about you, Ellen?" Brooke said, emphasizing the usage of Ellen's name. "What is your natural element? Golfing, I assume?"

"I like to golf, but it takes too much time. I am like you, Brooke. I love to work but taking 4-5 hours to play during the week is nearly impossible. I learned how to play from my ex-husband. When we were married, we played quite a bit. Mostly on the weekend, but if I don't play a lot, I don't play very well, and I try to do everything in my life well, and when I can't, I get frustrated." Stopping to take a sip of wine, Ellen continued, "Besides golf, I like walks in the park, reading, travel, and cooking a bit."

Ellen stopped, realizing that she probably shared more about her life with Brooke than she had with anyone new in a long time.

They sat in a brief awkward silence, broken up by Scott coming by to take their food order. After they ordered, another awkward silence fell, but Brooke broke it by asking, "So, Ellen, I am curious as to why you invited me to lunch. I appreciate it, of course, but did you have something specific you wanted to talk about?"

Ellen liked Brooke's directness. Another attribute they shared that Ellen picked up on.

"I did, Brooke. Dr. Finnegan and I enjoyed your visit with us, and we were wondering what you thought of our operation?"

"I was very impressed, but your approach seems edgy, counter-intuitive to what I have learned and followed as sound practice over the last several years. On the one hand, it seems like you are trying to improve and, in fact, challenge the existing processes, but on the other hand, it seems like you are doing something that in some way is, hmm," Brooke paused, searching for the word. She found it and said, "Ghoulish? I am not even sure if I am making any sense. Am I?"

Ellen laughed. "Perfect sense. You have summarized what many other medical professionals have told us and what we initially heard from our investors. Some of the investors are on the course now playing golf with Alex, and they probably are having the same conversation."

"The other thing I wondered was why the interest in me? I met Dr. Finnegan during a run at Forest Park, and he invited me for a tour, which frankly was more comprehensive than I thought it would be. More like a tour you would give to your investors. Then lunch with you now. All this seems like a lot of effort on your behalf. So, Ellen, why me?"

"All good questions, Brooke. But first, let's dispel any myths that the tour is what we would give our investors. Most are interested in the balance sheet and how much money they can make. To be honest with you, most of them are squeamish talking about death, or the medical jargon is way over their heads, and they avoid it to not look stupid in front of their colleagues. They usually just sit through a PowerPoint presentation, look at the financials, and if still not convinced, go through a little arm-twisting exercise which is what Alex is doing today."

"All well and good, Ellen, but you still did not answer my question. Why did I get all special treatment?"

Pausing a bit, both taking a few bites of their lunch, Ellen waited and answered, "You are a straightforward individual. We like that. You are also very smart and very talented at your job. We checked into your background before you came on the tour. Frankly, we would not have spent that much time with you in person on the tour if our inquiries about you did not come back so glowingly."

Now Brooke shifted a bit, uneasy in her chair. Maybe this was an interview.

Ellen continued, "We spent so much time with you before, during, and now after the tour because we view you as a peer, a colleague, or maybe something more. We are in the same business. We are getting a lifesaving organ from a donor to a recipient. You work for an institution, a hospital, and we are a private company, but our end goal is still the same. How we get there may be slightly different, and if you feel what we do is a bit *ghoulish*, or maybe underhanded and murky, that is natural since we are pushing the envelope for change, and change is sometimes messy and uncomfortable. Let me ask you something. What stood out to you most about our process, positively or negatively?"

After pausing to think about her answer, Brooke said, "I think the most positive takeaway was meeting the Ortel and Johnson families. See- ing how they interacted with each other, knowing that one of the families would lose a loved one, and the other family would benefit from that loss. While sadness still permeated the room, it seemed to me that there was a sense of optimism, maybe even a sense of togetherness that both families would lean on each other and become connected forever through the organ donation."

Nodding her head in agreement, Ellen said, "They will be connected forever, as are all families who share an organ. Over time we believe that the connection will improve the recipient's acceptance of the organ and help the Johnson family come to terms with Mr. Johnson's death and, in a way, see value in it. I know it's cliché, but sharing Mr. Johnson's virtue will extend Mr. Ortel's life."

Ellen continued, "Brooke, you don't know this about me, but I was adopted, and back then, it was very rare to have an open adoption. Most of the time, the adopted child never knew anything about their birth parents. I never knew my birth parents, and while I certainly could have researched them as I became an adult, I always thought it was an insult to my adoptive parents. Plus, I was a little scared of what I would find. I was not sure how I would feel if I found out my birth parents were great people who did not want me or could not care for me at the time or were horrible people who didn't deserve a child. Regardless of the cir- cumstances, there was and will always be an unknown connection to my birth parents and maybe siblings I might have out there. This connection, good or bad, will always be a missing piece of who I am. I believe what we do at the Transplant Center, connecting the soon-to-be dying with those who will go on and live, is filling a hole that needs filling for some people - like the holes filled with open adoptions. There is so much secrecy in the transplant process, and I think it is better to unmask everything and everyone in the process before the transplant occurs, not years after."

Brooke thought about what Ellen had just said and found herself silently in agreement with her. Brooke's best friend, Emma, was adopted, and she and Brooke had spent many summer evenings talking about the same thing. Emma was indecisive about finding her birth parents for all the reasons Ellen had mentioned. Brooke decided that she would broach the subject with Emma again this weekend.

Brooke snapped out of her silent thoughts about Emma when Ellen asked, "Brooke, you shared the positives you took from our tour. What about the negatives?"

Surprising Ellen, Brooke laughed. "Remember the movie *Fiddler on the Roof?*" Ellen nodded, though a bit confused by the analogy. "In the movie," Brooke went on, "there was the song *Matchmaker. Matchmaker, matchmaker, make me a match, find me a find, catch me a catch,*" Brooke quietly sang the words.

Now Ellen laughed a bit. "Yes, I remember the movie and song. Isn't the Muny in Forest Park doing *Fiddler on the Roof* this summer?"

Brooke thought about that for a second, returning to her chance encounter with Dr. Finnegan outside the Muny Box office. *Was Fiddler listed on the billboard? That would be odd,* she thought.

Not wanting to lose her concentration and thinking perhaps the glass of wine was making her foggy, Brooke wanted to make her point to Ellen. "What bothered me the most is that you are trying to play matchmaker in life and death, and that may be more God's domain than yours and Dr. Finnegan's. From what I understand, you are trying to bring a personal or human element into a process by introducing the donor and recipient families before the transplant. Transplants today are impersonal, clinical, data-driven, and anonymous, and, frankly, while the process is not perfect, it works pretty well," Brooke said, emphasizing the last point.

"You are right, Brooke. We are doing all those things because we think the outcomes are better for both the donor and recipient families. Time will tell if we are right. Based on our acceptance rate of transplanted organs, we will achieve ultimate patient satisfaction and happiness after the transplant. Because the recipient knows the donor family, they may see the psychological impact to the donor family seeing their loved one's organ alive in another individual."

Ellen went on. "Now, I debate whether we are trying step into God's role, or fate or whatever you want to call it about the matchmaking process of connecting a donor to a recipient. Rather than criticize us, it would be best if you questioned the blind faith you have in the medical industry and its rigid processes and procedures. I have been a doctor for a long time, and I know firsthand that the medical industry is slow to change unless they see a financial benefit from the change. The only reason CFOs or CEOs of the nation's medical centers care if their success rate in transplants or any procedures improves is if they can make more money. Or can use the improvement to tout in their marketing literature or with their large donors to raise more money."

Pausing for a second and slightly exasperated, Ellen said, "Really, you are a little naïve to think the institutions themselves care for the patient beyond how many dollars the patient is worth to them."

Regretting her shortness immediately with Brooke, Ellen tried to pull it back, but before she could speak, Brooke said, "Institutions may not care, Dr. Calabrese, but I care. My whole team cares. We cry when one of our patients gets a transplant, and we cry when they don't. We also silently pray for the donors, knowing they gave their lives so others can live. I think, Dr. Calabrese, perhaps you are the naïve one to think that medicine or those who administer medicine are cold and jaded." Uncomfortable silence enveloped the table. Ellen knew the mood would worsen as she saw Alex Finnegan approaching with the three golf partners and investors following him, all laughing, their game finished and ready to continue their good time at the bar.

Ellen caught Alex's eye with a quick warning to steer clear, but he either did not pick up on it or ignored it as he headed directly towards them. "Ellen, Brooke," he greeted them a little too loudly, indicating that their post-round drinks were not the first drinks they had today. "How are you, Brooke? Is Ellen a good host?"

"Hello, Dr. Finnegan," Brooke looked up. "Yes, we had a very nice lunch, and it is nice to see you again, but we were just finishing up."

"Please stay and join us for drinks on the patio."

"I wish I could, but I promised my parents I would help them at the restaurant tonight," Brooke said as she stood up. She quickly bid farewell to Dr. Calabrese and the investors and hastily exited the club.

Now suddenly understanding Ellen's cues, Alex directed his investors to the table on the patio. After motioning to Bill, the club's bartender, to take their drink orders, Alex turned to Ellen and said, "What the hell went on with her?"

"She is a very passionate, opinionated, and smart young woman, but she is not sold on our concept."

"The way she left, it seemed like she was also angry. Why? She is essential to us."

"Well, not sure she is angry at us, probably more me," Ellen said. "Maybe I am underestimating her, but I will turn her. Don't worry."

"Do it, Ellen. And quickly. Those three guys over there," looking towards the table on the patio, "won't be giving us our next big checks unless we can make vast improvements in our pipeline."

Ellen got up from her table and walked to the larger table outside to sit with Alex and the investors. As she sat down and made small talk, she thought about Brooke in the back of her mind. Yes, Brooke was going to need some special attention from her. It would be challenging and fun turning her, but she would turn her.

CHAPTER 27

After leaving the club, Brooke did not go to the restaurant, though she was sure her parents needed help. She returned to the hospital and her floor to check on her team and patients. It was common for Brooke to stop by, as her transplant patients and their families were on her mind 24/7, and whenever possible, even during off-hours, Brooke would visit and offer a bit of encouragement. During this visit, Brooke was going to provide encouragement and perhaps get some answers to questions she had for herself after her lunch with Dr. Calabrese.

While the lunch ended on a down note with Dr. Calabrese challenging and perhaps even ridiculing Brooke's thinking, Brooke was nothing if not reflective. She always looked for ways to grow, improve, and expand her thinking. She would not concede that Dr. Calabrese was right or wrong until she gathered more information. Brooke was not rigid or a pushover. She just had a process to follow to confirm her thinking, and the process this afternoon was to visit with her patients and get their thoughts if they were willing to give them.

Brooke visited the central nursing station to casually check in on her team and get an idea of any significant changes that had happened to any patients since she was last here. No changes. The same ten patients and their families were on the floor waiting for their lucky number to be called. At this stage, either their name was called to let them know they matched with an organ, or as days and hours passed, the grim realization that a match may not occur would begin to set in. The families then prepared for either a more extended hospital stay or, in the worst-case scenario, prepared for death. While she would try to stop and say hello to all her patients, she would not bother all of them for answers to her questions. She did not want to give them false hope that a new approach could be found or burden them more by asking them questions designed to satisfy her needs, not theirs.

She popped her head in just to offer a smile and words of encouragement to Mr. Andreas, Mrs. Pershing, and Mr. Konig. All patients had been in the hospital for about five days, awaiting a match for their lungs. They were not competing for the same lungs as they all had different blood types, antibodies, and body sizes. This competition issue arose quite a bit, mainly with the families who would get to know each other through laughter and tears in the waiting areas.

Brooke and her team knew it was only human nature that some family members or patients would wonder if they were getting passed by for a lung. Brooke knew, while not said out loud, that families would eye each other and wonder if their family member would lose out on a lung to a patient whose family they had gotten to know. This potential jealousy was why the hospital staff was so tight-lipped and protective about each patient and their history and records.

Although rare for two patients to have exact matching needs, because families did talk, patients with the same match criteria were housed in different parts of the floor with different waiting areas. This separation minimized the chances of an encounter or argument between families. Brooke also knew that while families suffered through this together, they were generally happy if they heard other patients got a transplant. Even though news of someone else getting a transplant gave those waiting a sense of despair, it also gave them hope.

Brooke popped into room 5110 to see Mrs. Martel. She was 65 and had been in the hospital waiting for lungs due to COPD. In most COPD cases, smoking was the cause, but Mrs. Martel did not smoke a day in her life. She was from a farm family in rural Illinois, primarily raising pigs, and the years spent inhaling the dust from the pens took its toll on Mrs. Martel. She was a perfect candidate for a lung transplant and was otherwise healthy. Her husband, Richard, of nearly 40 years, stayed by her side as much as Covid protocol would allow. Many days and nights, the Martels would FaceTime their children and grandchildren to keep their spirits up.

Brooke knocked before entering and, as she did, saw the Martel's doing their favorite pastime: the New York Times crossword puzzle.

As she looked up and lowered her reading glasses, Mrs. Martel smiled at Brooke and exclaimed,

"Just what we need! A young person with more brains than we have. Brooke, what is a seven-letter word for pecs and abs?"

Brooke thought a minute and said confidently, "Muscles."

"Brains and beauty," Richard said to Brooke, always a bit of a flirt, even at his advanced age of 70.

"That fits!" said Mrs. Martel, the official crossword puzzle scribe, as she had the better handwriting.

"I thought you worked the morning shift. Why are you here now, my dear? Friday night and to visit us? A beautiful woman like yourself must have something more exciting to do."

"Nothing more exciting than seeing my two favorite pig farmers," Brooke laughed. It was a theme of an ongoing joke as Mr. Martel promised that if insurance did not cover their bill, they would pay Brooke and the medical staff in pigs.

"How are you doing, Mrs. Martel?" Brooke asked.

"Feeling good. Well, as good as I can feel, but waiting to get the call so I can get out of this hospital and see our kids and grandkids. I also need to tend to my garden. I'm sure Richard hasn't been keeping that up."

Richard Martel, slightly hard of hearing and refusing to wear hearing aids, barely looked up, either because he was not paying attention or did not hear the comment. He had taken the crossword puzzle from his wife, intently staring at it.

"Do you mind if I can break you two away from your crossword puzzle to ask you a few questions?"

"Sure, Brooke, ask away," Mrs. Martel said, adding a little louder than usual to ensure Richard heard her. "Richard put that dang crossword puzzle down for a second. Brooke wants to ask us some questions."

"Why are you yelling?" Richard yelled back. "I'm right here."

Brooke let their temporary outburst of false anger settle for a minute and stifled a smile and light laugh. She knew the Martels loved each other and cherished her relationship with them. Brooke knew their love came from daily devotion to one another and their animated banter because of Richard's lack of hearing or attention. She saw in them a life that she hoped to have with her partner communicating a lifetime of memories with an eye roll, a shrug, or even a fake outburst of anger. Her parents were like the Martel's. Their marriage survived and thrived through verbal and non-verbal communication, working together daily in the restaurant.

Her thoughts of her parents, the Martel's, and even her future, what-ever that may be, were what drove her to care so much about her job. Lately, she began questioning if she was doing everything possible to help her transplant patients survive and thrive. They may be physically only with her at the hospital for two or three weeks as they were preparing for and recovering from a transplant, but thoughts and memories of them and how they were doing lasted forever. She also met many extended family members and thought of the toll this process had on them.

Clearing her head, Brooke asked the Martels, "Please bear with me, but I would like to get your opinion on something I recently experienced. Remember that this has nothing to do with the hospital, the transplant process, or the care you are getting. It is more a personal request to help me evaluate something."

"Sounds like a caper," Richard replied.

"Shut up, Richard. Let the girl talk," shot back Mrs. Martel but with a smile on her face.

Brooke continued, "Thanks. As you know, during the transplant pro-cess, we apply your transplant vitals and requirements against the UNOS national database, in your case, lungs, and if there is a match and your transplant score places you on the top of the list, then you get the lungs. Throughout the process, you do not know who donated the lungs, and you may or may not have a choice to find out who donated them. That is how the process works for all transplants in the United States, except for living transplant donors who donate kidneys where a family member may donate one of their kidneys to another."

The Martels nodded in agreement, so Brooke continued.

"What if you had the chance to meet your donor and their family before they passed away? Would that be something you think you would do?"

The Martels thought in silence for a minute, with finally Richard asking, "Is that even possible?"

"Well, in theory, yes, if a person who has agreed to donate their lungs upon death and the death could be anticipated a few weeks in advance. But in the case of sudden death, obviously no," Brooke answered.

"It would seem weird to meet the person who is going to die so you can live," Mrs. Martel chimed in.

"What if the donor's family wanted to meet the possible recipients so they could feel good about where the donor's organs were going? What if you spent some time together in a pre-transplant health care facility where you got to know the donor? Perhaps your families got to know each other, and you could ask any question of them and them of you?" Brooke asked them both.

Again, about thirty seconds of silence before Richard Martel answered with, "I know I am not the one getting the transplant, but if I did ever need one, yes, I think I would like to know something about the person whose organ I am getting. And I would want them and their family to know something about me. I would want them to believe that I was a good guy, not a scoundrel who would waste the precious gift they had given me. If the roles were reversed, and I was donating an organ, I would want to know where and to whom my organ was going."

Mrs. Martel sat quietly in her thoughts.

"Mrs. Martel, what do you think?" Brooke turned and asked her.

"Well, in one way, the impersonal and anonymous nature of the process blocks your emotions that someone died so I could live. Not putting a name or face or seeing a person's family seems to help me accept what is going to happen, but after I got the transplant, I would start wondering about the donor. What their life was like; how their family is coping with their loss. So, while I initially thought the idea was kind of weird, even creepy, maybe meeting the donor before the transplant would give me more peace of mind after the transplant."

As Brooke and the Martel's thought a bit more in silence, Brooke looked down at her hospital-issued cell phone, which had just pinged.

"Can we do that? Can we meet our possible donor?" Richard asked.

Looking up, Brooke looked at both of the Martels. "It's too late, unfortunately, for Mrs. Martel," she said.

Startled at what Brooke had just said, Richard and Mrs. Martel looked at each other, fearing the worst, but if they had turned to Brooke instead, they would have noticed a smile beginning to cross her face as she texted something into her cell phone.

Before they could turn to her, Brooke said, "Well, I hope you two have picked out some nice pigs for payment because you will be out of this hospital in about two weeks. You matched! You will receive a new lung in the next 4-5 hours."

With that, Brooke got up from her chair to hug Richard and Mrs. Martel, who had processed the news and began crying. Mrs. Martel whispered in Brooke's ear, "Now I wish I had met the donor."

Brooke, wishing them luck with a tear in her eye and some clarity in her thinking, left the room as it began to fill with the team on duty who would prepare Mrs. Martel for surgery.

CHAPTER 28

Vinnie could not stop thinking about Frank at a stoplight on his way home. His bad luck. His weakening condition. His time left on earth if he did not get the transplant. He was startled out of his thoughts by a horn behind him. The light turned green and had been green long enough for the driver of the honking car not only to honk but also to pull around Vinnie, yelling out of his window, "Wake up, asshole!"

Vinnie just smiled and waved at the angry driver, his standard response to hopefully diffuse road rage. While Vinnie certainly would use a few expletives on a bad golf shot, when interacting with people on the road, he thought it best to keep his cool. He always wondered how people felt expressing such anger, usually at strangers. Did they feel bad about it? Did they feel remorse? Vinnie would never take the bait because he did not want his day ruined by someone who could not manage their emotions. Life was too short to get angry over minor things, and knowing what Frank was going through reinforced that to Vinnie.

As he got nearer to his home, his mind drifted back to Frank, so much so that he did not notice the light changing to red. He braked quickly, only to stop within feet of the car in front of him. He immediately expected a middle finger raised in his direction or the driver's hand gesturing outside their window, but he got no reaction from the driver, who he could now see was an older woman. With his heart rate slowing down from his near-crash, Vinnie noticed writing on the back window of the yellow, late model Toyota in front of him:

Please Help. I need a kidney transplant.

Please text me: 314-555-9878

Vinnie just stared at the message and thought, *how can this be that in 2021, in the United States, supposedly the most prosperous country in the world and with the best health care system, this woman must beg strangers for a kidney?* Vinnie did not know much about transplants and was learning quite a lot from Frank, but he thought kidneys should be easy to get as he knew that living donors from family member to family member were possible.

Perhaps this woman had no family, or worse, her family refused to help. He wanted to jump out of his truck and talk to her. However, he knew with carjackings happening at an alarming rate in St. Louis and all over the country, his movement toward the car might startle her or, worse: injure him if she was carrying a handgun. He tried to wave to her through his windshield, but she did not look up. As the light turned green, she turned left while Vinnie went straight. He quickly grabbed his cell phone to snap a photo of her car's back window and phone number. He was unsure what he hoped to learn from her or if he would call her, but maybe he could learn something or even help in some way if he contacted her.

Vinnie got to his house a bit shaken, more so from the encounter with the woman needing a kidney versus the earlier asshole yelling at him. He headed for the kitchen and turned on his Keurig for a cup of coffee. He also turned on his computer to learn more about the state of transplants in the United States. Vinnie, of course, had an accessible expert with his ex-wife, Ellen, who was now the Chief Medical Officer of the Transplant Center. Perhaps he would reach out to her, but in his youth and still today, Vinnie loved to read and research. He would read on any subject, any time of the day. As a teenager, his friends chastised him because, at parties, Vinnie would often find a corner and grab a book or magazine to read rather than engage in the regurgitation of the same conversations and boasts that would take place day in and day out with his friends. His reply to his friends who would tease him unmercifully was, "learning is interesting, and when you guys say something interesting, I am all ears." His friends did not realize that while girls always gravitated toward the good-looking guys at parties, a few would find his behavior a bit eccentric and wander over to investigate this shy bookworm. Vinnie got many phone numbers that way, but he kept that secret from his friends. His love of reading was how he first met Ellen and, in some ways, how he also lost her.

But today, his companion for his online research was his stray black cat, who he named Finn after he found him and his litter mates several years ago as kittens, dumped on the banks of the nearby Meramec River. Today, with intrusions by Finn, who would take his turn jabbing at the keyboard, Vinnie would learn all he could about transplants. Linking to Google, Vinnie typed in 'transplants,' which gave him many choices on the search page. He went to www.organdonor.gov and found the main page had an easy-to-read dashboard. He knew some general stats for transplants as he was an active blood donor at the Red Cross Blood, and the material he read there reinforced the need to consider being an organ donor. But these stats startled him on how much of a problem still existed with transplants.

He read that a person is added to the transplant waiting list every 9 minutes. Over 6000 people per year and 17 people a day die without getting the needed transplant. One hundred seven thousand people are currently on the transplant waiting list in the United States. One donor could save eight lives with the organs available for transplant. It seemed to Vinnie that in the supply and demand business, transplants were all demand and not enough supply. Thinking back to the plea for help he saw listed on the woman's car, he researched kidneys a bit more and realized why she was so desperate.

There was almost four times the number of kidneys needed than available donors. It was by far the organ most in-demand and the least amount of supply. Lungs also had issues because of Covid, but they had much less need and a closer balance of supply and demand.

However, while the data on the website was relatively current, Vinnie wondered how Covid would affect lung transplant supply and demand. Covid was causing a higher rate of people having lung damage that, in many cases, needed to be saved by a lung transplant. Additionally, the long-term viability of a lung transplant patient was much lower than other organs. *Perhaps,* Vinnie thought, *the demand was lower because those who needed them decided against the operation as the outcome was not that promising as most lung transplants only live eight years on average.* Vinnie knew Frank wanted to have the procedure regardless of the risk and long-term outcome as he was relatively young, just under 60 and had children just starting their lives as young adults and a few grandchildren that he wanted to watch grow up. Frank was also a fighter, never giving up regardless of how much life sometimes held him back. Vinnie thought God owed Frank a lung. He was owed a long life. Vinnie knew he wanted to help Frank in any way possible but did not know where to start.

Maybe talking to Ellen would be a good start as she was the most knowledgeable person he knew. He placed a call to her and got her voice mail, which he expected as Ellen never answered her phone the first time, both because of screening calls and preferring to be texted. So rather than leave a message, he texted her to call him about Frank. He knew that adding Frank's name to the reason for the text would prompt a quicker response from Ellen as she was deeply fond of Frank and knew that he was sick. Ellen might not have entirely known the extent of Frank's situation unless she had gotten more updates directly from Frank and Sue than the scarce ones Vinnie occasionally provided.

CHAPTER 29

⁓✦⁓

While not admitting it to herself or her fellow cops, Detective Simon did prioritize the energy she put into investigating certain murder cases. The case of William Thomson would receive most of her energy despite it being the most recent killing on her overloaded caseload. While never discussed in police protocol, she knew her direct superiors and the movers and shakers of St. Louis politicians, business leaders, and sports team owners wanted the Thomson case solved. It involved an innocent person doing something all of St. Louis could relate to, taking a grandchild to a Cardinals game.

Downtown St. Louis was experiencing continuous white flight, as the city's population had been consistently dropping since the mid-1950s, becoming, for the first time, a city with more non-white residents than not. Along with the white flight, businesses were fleeing the city and the entire region. Recently a major law firm, usually a bedrock of business tenants in downtown St. Louis, had decided to move most of its 300 attorneys to the western suburbs. Any attempts to keep corporations in the city stalled whenever a heinous crime, like the murder of Bill Thomson, occurred.

They blamed Covid and a reduced need for office space due to the work-from-home phenomena that had taken place over the last year. Still, it was no coincidence that they decided to put their building on the market weeks after one of their young female partners was accosted, then murdered in a carjacking in the law firm's garage. Detective Simon was not assigned that case, but since the Thomson case and that case both involved a carjacking, she would be sure to compare notes with the investigating detective.

Reviewing videos from the parking lot and street cameras in the Thomson case, she could begin to see the crime unfolding. It was worse than watching a horror movie since she knew the ending. She saw Mr. Thomson and his grandson happily walking down 7th street from Busch Stadium. Both talked very animatedly, and Mr. Thomson held his grandson's hand to ensure he kept up the pace. Detective Simon sensed that based on his body language and the way his eyes canvassed the surroundings as they walked, Mr. Thomson had his radar up as he knew the possible risks of leaving the game early. The cameras from Paddy O's bar picked them up, passing the outdoor patio, and then the street cameras picked them up, turning into the parking lot where the crime occurred just north of Kilroy's Bar. Simon then turned to the footage of cameras from Nestle-Purina's parking lot, west of the crime scene, and street cameras east, south, and north within a two-block radius. She assumed the suspects were casing a general area around the parking lots and would need a clear view of their victims and any parking lot security, police presence, or people gathering.

Since she did not see any sign of the possible assailants on the cameras that picked up Mr. Thomson, she rewound the footage in 15-minute intervals. She assumed the suspects were loitering in the area looking for victims and that this crime, while a crime of opportunity, was planned to some degree. She got a hit after about 20 minutes when she saw two young black males standing underneath the railroad trestle, just north of the Gas House Bar and Grill and south of Kilroy's. Due to the graininess of the footage, Detective Simon couldn't determine their exact age. From this vantage point, the two males would be able to see multiple parking lots, as well as stragglers leaving early from Busch Stadium. While unsure, she had a hunch these two were the same two seen taunting her from a distance after she had wrapped up the crime scene. She remembered them running down 7th street south before stopping to talk and then getting in a car that had pulled up to the side of the road just before the I-44 and I-55 on-ramp off 7th street.

She remembered that encounter and, at the time, found it odd that while running away, they had a specific goal: to intersect with the white car. The driver in the vehicle knew these men as no one leaving the game would stop and talk to these guys unless they knew them. That got her thinking, so she decided to look farther back in time at the video. Looking at the same camera footage that picked them up initially, she went back another 15 minutes, then another, until she found what she was looking for. A white, late-model Audi had appeared on 7th street at approximately 7:00 p.m. when the arriving baseball crowd mainly had thinned from the streets in a hurry to get into the stadium before the first pitch. The car pulled over on 7th street near the Eat Rite Diner, where Detective Simon had first eyed the men. In the video exiting the car, she saw the two men. They left the car, and after a brief conversation through the driver's side window, they headed north to the spot where she had seen them on camera observing the parking lots. The car, however, did not go far after dropping off the men. It just moved farther south on 7th near the Rock House bar.

Not close enough to see what the two men would be doing but close enough, as it turns out, to intersect with them after the crime was committed. Detective Simon knew she had to look at cameras closer to the Rock House bar to see if she could get a plate on the Audi.

Turning the video footage off for a minute, she thought about what pieces she had on video. She had the victim, Mr. Thomson. She had the two men on the street before and after the crime was committed. She had a car transporting the men within a block of the crime scene, and she had her interaction possibly with the same two men after the crime scene running away, but then meeting the same white Audi as they fled down 7th. What she did not have on camera were the two men, or anyone committing the crime of attempted carjacking, then shooting and murdering Mr. Thomson. The only actual eyewitness was his 6-year-old grandson. She did not want to talk to the little boy if she did not need to, as he would surely be traumatized, but he was the only witness, for now.

Taking a deep breath and looking to clear her mind, she casually looked over the other unsolved cases on her docket. None of the crimes seemed connected as they happened in various parts of town with different seemingly unrelated victims and causes of death. But still, she pulled up the files to see if any new information was added or witnesses found. Most of these cases were getting close to a month old, nearly stone-cold in her line of work.

A meth head overdosing on Olive Street in the middle of the day. No connection. A random hit and run of a bike rider in Forest Park. No connection, but she did remember she wanted to investigate her overzealous witness, Vinnie Calabrese, a bit more. He seemed like an odd character. The shooting of William Burroughs was drug or revenge related with witnesses but none who could identify the shooter, despite nearly 20 people in the same vicinity as the victim when the crime occurred. She was about the close the file when she reread the anonymous tip on the hotline about seeing a newer model white Audi dropping off two young males near the house minutes before the killing of William Burroughs. Detective Simon's experience told her not to get too excited about a similar brand car being seen in two crimes a few weeks apart. Especially since the crimes were in different parts of the city and the assumed motives and victims were completely unrelated. Still, it would have to be something that she needed to follow up on, which made her job so difficult, as any clue required follow-up, and that took time and resources, both of which she was short on as the police department was woefully understaffed.

Her phone rang as she sat thinking about the two white Audis and if there was any connection between them and the two crimes. Answering, she was greeted by a familiar voice. "Rhonda, how the hell are you?" said Detective Angie Sullivan, a friend and peer of Rhonda's. Rhonda replied, "I am fine, Angie. Great to hear from you. It has been too long. What do I owe the pleasure?"

"You mean besides giving you grief because you have disappeared from the face of the earth, and I have not seen you at McGurk's in a long time. I assume a new man has got your attention, right Rhonda?" she laughed, a full hearty laugh that Rhonda loved to hear and now needed to hear.

"You can say it's a man, Angie, multiple men, but they are a bit stiff and not in a good way." Rhonda then let out a laugh of her own, joined on the other end of the line by Angie, who immediately got the joke. They both could give and take the raunchy humor as that was part of their job in the male-dominated environment in which they worked.

With the laughter subsiding and both Detectives knowing they could zing each other with one-liners all day, Rhonda broke the pattern and asked, "Well, let's hear it, lady. You called me. What's on your mind?"

"Carjackings," Angie Sullivan replied. "In case you don't realize it, we have a bit of an epidemic of carjackings in the city," she added sarcastically. "I understand you are working a bad one with the old man. What was his name, Thomson? An attempted carjack and murder while walking back from a Cards' game with his grandson."

"Yep. Not sure it was a carjacking attempt, but it's a bad one, and it has gotten the attention of City Hall and Civic Progress. They want it solved quickly to reassure the public it was not some random act and that the crown jewel of downtown, Cardinals games, are perfectly safe to attend. So, are you calling about that case because I could use the help?" Rhonda asked.

"Well, maybe I can help you, and you can help me. I am assigned to lead a task force to see if there is any common theme among carjackings in different city quadrants. We feel the carjackers work in the same general area as there are plenty of opportunities, and they know all the escape routes. We think kids do most, and I hate to call them that when they are packing some pretty heavy weaponry, and most done for the gang initiation rite of passage or just kicks."

Rhonda agreed with what Angie was saying, as it was a fact that most carjacked cars ended up abandoned a few miles away, beat up from joy riding but not stripped of parts, or sent to chop shops. These kids, as Angie called them, were riding around in vehicles worth 40K or more, and the only value the carjackers got was what they stole from the car or the victim's purse or wallet. It made no sense financially, but the carjackers were not on the path to an Ivy League education. But the carjackings had taken an ominous turn as the rite of passage for gang initiation often added murder to the plan. Adding to the carnage, more citizens were also packing heat, and while police constantly reinforced that the victim should hand over the keys and run, increased shootings occurred when the victim decided to fire away. Sometimes it worked. Sometimes it did not, but the problem was not going away. The problem was only getting worse.

"Rhonda, do you have anything solid on the possible assailants in the Thomson case?" Angie asked.

"Maybe. I reviewed street and business videos, and I can confirm that two men, maybe a third, not sure of age, were near the scene an hour before the incident occurred. I also had by chance an ugly encounter with them after I arrived on the scene and was wrapping up."

"What kind of encounter?" Angie asked.

"You know the usual kind. Fuck you, po-po. Gesturing fingers, grabbing their crotches, for God knows why, language you wouldn't kiss your mother, father, sister, or brother with. Just another glorious day basking in the respect we get on the job," Rhonda sighed.

"Anything else?" asked Angie.

"Anyway, on video, I saw the two immature assholes, after being dropped off by a white Audi, lingering around the parking lots where the murder occurred, about an hour or so before it went down. Then about 30 minutes after the shooting occurred, and after we exchanged pleasantries, I saw them running down 7th street, stopping and getting into a car that, if I were pressed on it, while I could not positively confirm a make, I would say was the same white Audi."

Angie asked, "Do you think you could recognize these fine men if I showed you some footage that we have of recent carjackings?"

"Possibly. What do you have?" asked Rhonda.

"You remember the case a few weeks ago in the garage of the law firm, McConnell and McGrath? Well, we have some excellent video of our young future Rhoades Scholars shooting the victim, taking her car, and driving about 100 yards before it stalled out because it was a stick shift, and they could not drive it. Of course, they could have had the victim give them a lesson in driving a stick shift, but she was 100 yards away dying after they shot her," said Detective Sullivan, with anger and sarcasm in her voice.

Rhonda chimed in, finishing what she knew were Angie's thoughts, "So these guys, who may be 17 but will never make it to 25, assaulting and killing the victims. In both instances, they left the car but for different reasons. Both crimes were within one mile of each other. Around the same time of evening, when the Cardinals were playing. Right?"

"Right on all counts," Angie responded. "So, can I get you interested enough to come by and look at some video and, if you do, drinks on me after?"

"Ok, but let's allocate a little more time. I want to review some different videos. I am assuming that since your garage cameras had such a clear view of the crime, you did not need to go back in time to see if anything else of interest occurred?"

"Yeah, that is right. We saw the assailants come out of the stairwell in the garage, assault and kill the victim, try to drive away, then run like hell when the car stalled. We assume we have it all since it seems straightforward. What am I missing?" Angie inquired.

"Well, maybe nothing, but I would love to see if my friend in the white Audi might have shown up before or after the carjacking. Can you pull the video in 15-minute increments inside the garage and on the street where the troubled youths might have left the garage? I would like to go back at least an hour from when the crime was committed and then look at some street angles within 10 minutes of when the car stalled and they ran for it. And my dear Angie, if I happen to see a white Audi, I will buy you dinner."

"It's a date," said Angie. "Come by the precinct tomorrow around 4:00 p.m., and we'll spend a few hours on this. Looking forward to seeing you, my friend, and maybe we can put some of these misguided youths on the path to salvation in one of our fine penal institutions."

CHAPTER 30

D r. Ellen James-Calabrese and Dr. Alex Finnegan sat together in the board room of the Transplant Center. They knew they had a problem. They sat in silence after debating the solution to it, even though it might compromise all ethics they swore to as doctors.

After spending all day wooing investors, then several days later, in this very board room, presenting them with the business case and financial return of the Arch City Transplant Center, they had succeeded. The investors had opened their checkbooks and offered to provide millions of dollars of funding to make the Transplant Center the nation's and maybe even the world's leading alternative in the transplant business.

Of course, the investors expected a very healthy return on their investment, one that Alex Finnegan's ego had no doubt he could deliver. While not saying it out loud, he knew that this moment was the culmination of his brilliance, drive, and risk-taking over the last 20 years, combining his medical and business education. He was already wealthy and successful, a true one-percenter, but he wanted more. He wanted power over people, but the one person he had to convince was Dr. Calabrese sitting next to him, casting doubts on his plans.

He hired Ellen to be his Chief Medical Officer in part because he wanted her to run the medical aspect of The Center. At the same time, he handled the business end as his goal was to monetize, quickly and in significant sums, The Center's success. While he valued her feedback and counterarguments on his vision, he always felt that she would see things his way at the end of the day. However, he knew an argument was brewing about how The Center would make the revenue numbers in the timeframe Alex promised the investors.

It had been several hours since the last investor presentation concluded. Ellen got up from her chair to pour herself and Alex two glasses of Blanton's bourbon in preparation for a long night of intense debate on what they had just promised the investors.

"Alex, let's think this through. What you promised the investors you could deliver may not be possible because much of it is out of our control."

Alex promised the investors that The Center would grow revenue exponentially over the next five years by increasing the number of transplants done each year ten-fold from its current pace of 60. With each transplant worth approximately $250,000 to The Center, Alex had committed that The Center's revenue would grow from $15,000,000 to $150,000,000 million per year. Additionally, Alex laid out plans to expand the concept beyond St. Louis and into five more major metros that would support large regional swathes of the country. He had picked Cleveland, Kansas City, Louisville, Memphis, and Detroit as his expansion cities, all with similar supply and demand problems as St. Louis. He had outlined the total costs of operation, including land development, building construction or purchase, staffing, marketing, etc. All in, Alex had not only told but promised the investors that The Transplant Center would be a two-billion-dollar business in five years, and each of them would, in return, triple their investment and make hundreds of millions of dollars. As Ellen sat and listened to Alex's presentation, she thought, as she and done so many times, that *he was either a madman or a genius*, but listening to him rant about his plans, she was leaning toward madman. Of course, when the investors turned to her for confirmation of the plans, Ellen dutifully agreed wholeheartedly with Alex as she would see her stock in The Center be worth over $100 million if the plans all came to fruition.

Finally, Alex responded to Ellen and said, "Let's talk about the problems we are trying to solve here. We are trying to improve what we both agree to be an inefficient way of creating more donor supply and better efficiency and success in handling transplants, both from a medical, governmental, and cultural perspective. Correct?"

"Yes," Ellen quietly said as she began to soften from the long day catching up to her or from the Blanton's she was drinking.

"To do this, we must change our laws, values, and culture, and we also must respect that each person has a choice over their bodies, in life, and death. All of this is well overdue. Without these changes, thousands of people in the U.S. die each year without getting an organ."

Sitting up in her chair to make a more forceful point of her disagreement on the subject, Ellen said."Yes, but these changes you are trying to achieve should be done in Washington by our elected politicians whose job it is to make laws that benefit our citizens,"

"Oh, Ellen, for a smart woman, you are so naïve. Do you believe our politicians can get their heads out of their asses long enough to make laws that will benefit our vision and do it in our lifetime? This subject of transplants, the subject of how we die, is fraught with so many competing interests like insurance companies, religious leaders, and the medical profession, each fighting tooth, and nail to promote what they believe is right. What they believe, they have a moral say over. The only way to get what we need is to push the envelope. Get the people who believe in our vision and want choice on our side. When we do, we will generate enough cash that these competing interests will see how well we will line their pockets by supporting us. Then they will make the laws. It's all about money first, Ellen. The donors, the recipients, the special interests will do our bidding when they see how it will affect them financially."

"Well, you are certainly pushing the envelope on this, but I don't like the optics of the groups you are initially targeting," Ellen said.

"Hell, if, I mean when, this works, I will be a conquering hero to those groups, locally and nationally. The left and right will both love me because I support the individual's choice and the exclusion of government in that choice. They will also love me because I will be pouring money into people in the inner city, which may reduce crime and clean up the cities. I could run for damn President when this succeeds."

"Jesus, Alex. You have gone from a smart, confident, and successful businessperson to an egomaniac, and a dangerous one at that." Ellen shot back, wondering what happened to the Alex Finnegan she had admired so much.

"We are doing nothing dangerous or illegal. Eight states have passed laws supporting choice in death, and we will take advantage of that momentum and push the envelope on this, even if it finds us in court. As far as the other strategy, the insurance companies have been selling life insurance policies for hundreds of years and making billions. We are just putting a new spin on it and are giving the poor a chance to cash in and benefit from their misfortune for a change. Our lawyers have signed off on it, our investors are ok with it, and frankly, you need to get your head around this as well, as this is what we need to do," Alex said to Ellen with a tone that was more forceful than she was comfortable hearing.

Ellen pushed back, "I have heard all these points before, and I guess in theory, what we are doing may be legal or at least defendable in court, though I question if ethically in the court of public opinion. But logistically, how do you think we can pull this off?"

"You don't need to worry about how we will do it. I already have things in motion. You just need to handle the caseload of donors when I deliver them to our doorstep. I can give you one hundred million reasons why you need to do that."

Ellen hated that Alex used the huge payout as motivation. Ellen, like Alex, was very successful, though she did not have the burning desire to achieve power through massive wealth as Alex did. When Alex first approached her for the opportunity, she was both flattered and intrigued with the concept because she believed it would improve people's lives and increase the number of people getting successful transplants. But the monster that The Center and Alex had become was ravenous and needed to be fed. "Ok, while I disagree with some of your vision and how you plan to accomplish it, I want you to know that my job as Chief Medical Officer is the medical side of the business. My job is to ensure we treat the families well and that the transplants have a high degree of success. Your job is how we create the supply and demand to make you and your investors happy and richer. I prefer to be kept out of that side of the business as much as possible."

"I will keep you, if possible, on a need-to-know basis, so you have some degree of deniability, but you are into this deeper than you want to believe, and if you want out, you can resign now."

Ellen said nothing but got up and poured herself a little more Blanton's. This time she did not pour Alex a glass. She leaned against the conference room bar and thought for a minute. Finally, she said, "Well, first, quit trying to bully me by forcing me to accept your terms or resign. I deserve more respect than that. You would not even be able to manage the medical side of the business had you not brought me on. You know it, and I know it. So, about your resignation ultimatum, screw you, Alex. Secondly, I will do my job and hire medical personnel to ensure we improve the lives of our patients and their families. That is my goal, and that is what I plan to focus on."

Now Alex was silent, thinking about the fire in Ellen. It attracted him to her professionally, and he could not deny it, sometimes sexually. But Alex believed in the motto, don't shit where you eat, and as good-looking and sexy as Ellen was at her age, Alex liked younger women, and right now, he was thinking of one that he needed and wanted in his business, and perhaps in his bed.

"Ok, Ellen," he said. "I respect your position, and it is good to have some separation within the operation. Let's work on building your staff up because next week, you will have $30 million in your budget to expand your medical resources."

Putting her glass down, Ellen said, "Lots of work to do, starting tomorrow. See you, Alex."

Alex stayed in the boardroom after Ellen left. Although the 4th floor of the building was empty for nearly three hours, Alex instinctively got up and looked outside the boardroom to ensure no staff was staying late, and the cleaning crew was not around. He closed the door and sat down to make two calls, one business and one personal.

"Kenny, Alex. Yeah, we finished with the investor pitches. Yep. We got what we wanted. Ellen was her typical pain in the ass, but she will come around. Let's meet tomorrow around noon to go over your end of this. See you then."

He then made his call. "Hi Brooke, Alex Finnegan. Guess I got your voice mail. Probably too late to call back now, but if you get the chance, give me a call over the next couple of days. Thanks."

With the two calls placed and with silence in the room and building, Alex poured himself the last of the Blanton's. Sipping it, overlooking the late summer sun setting west of Forest Park, he thought to himself smugly how he always gets his way, eventually.

Talking to no one in particular, he toasted his reflection in the window. "Screw being President. I want to become king of the fucking world!"

CHAPTER 31

At noon, Alex went to the Art Museum in Forest Park. As he had done since he started The Center, he met with his medical school roommate, colleague, and friend for life, Dr. Kenny Thorton. While professionally, Kenny lost his medical license, partly due to Alex's negligence and arrogance, he would always be the best doctor Alex would ever know. Kenny and Alex met under the namesake statue of the city of St. Louis, a 20-foot-high King Louis IX that overlooked the expanse of Forest Park, the lakes to the east, and guarded the doors of the Art Museum to the west. Alex saw Kenny working his way leisurely on the paths encircling Grand Basin and up Art Hill. Kenny leisurely walked as if he had not a care in the world, and in a way, he did not. Alex took good care of him financially after he lost his medical license, giving him special assignments here and there to ensure the money was off the books. That money was much more than Kenny could make as a doctor. Alex owed that to Kenny.

"Kenny boy, how the hell are you?" Alex smiled and held out his arms to hug Kenny as he made his way up the last few feet of the Hill towards the statue.

"If I were any better, I would be living your life," Kenny replied.

"Well, Kenny, that's good to hear, but we both know that your life and mine are about to get much better."

"And richer," Kenny added.

It was an unusually cool and less humid summer day in St. Louis, so they decided rather than spend their usual hour in the Art Museum, they would just walk through the park, discussing, out in the open air, a very private conversation. They headed from the museum south about 500 yards towards the north entrance of the St. Louis Zoo.

"Ok, Alex. Based on your call last night, it sounded like your presentation went well. The investors are in, and even Ellen got the memo to get on the program."

"Yeah, I got guys giving millions of dollars to me, and they were easier than Ellen to convince. Honestly, I love the woman, but sometimes she can be a pain in the ass," Alex said.

"The fiery ones are worth it," Kenny commented. Alex knew he wasn't commenting on Ellen's business acumen or demeanor but her, as Kenny had always had a thing for Ellen ever since she divorced, in Kenny's mind, that loser of a husband, Vinnie. Ellen questioned Alex about his friendship with Kenny many times. If only Kenny knew that Ellen had nothing but disgust for him, he would give up his absurd fantasy of hooking up with her.

For his part, Alex knew that keeping Kenny in the shadows, far away from Ellen, was essential to keep this operation on track. One sight of Kenny with Alex at The Center and Ellen would quickly blow a gasket and persecute Alex.

"Kenny, let's not worry about Ellen right now. In fact, as the President of TTWC Life Insurance Company, you have a lot on your plate."

Kenny liked that Alex had appointed him President of the company, even though Kenny knew Alex would always call the shots. It gave Kenny some sense of respectability and self-worth. "So, when do I get a golf club membership and a better company car than your used Audi?" Kenny laughed.

"Hell, if this goes as planned, you can buy a whole damn golf course all for yourself, and you won't be driving my hand-me-downs."

Since Alex had about 30 minutes before he needed to get back to The Center, he wanted an update from Kenny on the progress of TTWC.

"So far, we are in excellent shape with the staffing of our localized and neighborhood agents," Kenny said. "We have ten agents working in the city's northern neighborhoods, another three in midtown, and five in the south corridor neighborhoods. I aim to get 30 total to account for planned and unplanned defection."

"That's good. How are the presentations going? Are we finding we are more successful in larger groups or working one-on-one in the neighborhoods?"

"Both really," Kenny went on. "We have found that presentations to church groups and community centers create wider exposure as more are hearing our message, and then when we do smaller groups or 1:1 sessions, people seem to have heard of our concept. Barber shops, funerals, pawn shops, check cashing, gun shops, we seem to do very well writing a policy on the spot. I would say we have a conversion rate of around 10%, but I hope to get that up to 20% when the agents start seeing some cold cash in their hands.

"That is great, Kenny. And no suspicion? No, nosy grandmothers sticking their noses in our business?" Alex asked.

"None so far. And no FBI, local cops, SEC, or any regulatory authority have rung my doorbell. You know, Alex, you have always been one smart, sneaky son of a bitch, ever since medical school, but this scam might be your best one yet," said Kenny.

Alex smiled at that. He knew he was one smart and sneaky son of a bitch, but he also knew Kenny matched him in both traits, and since getting his medical license revoked, Kenny had the added motivation of a big "get even" chip on his shoulders. Nothing like a very motivated person who needs the money to get the job done.

With the update done, Alex handed Kenny a backpack with $200,000 in it. The money was to pay Kenny his share, pay his agents their commissions, and pay off any life insurance claims to the families when the time was right.

"Kenny, this should last you about a month unless business gets too good, and based on the trends, it looks like we will have a great summer of hate, so business should be strong," Alex laughed. "If you need more before our meeting next month, just give me the signal, and I will meet you sooner than planned. Same place and time. Oh, and Kenny, be careful with that money. Your agents aren't exactly trustworthy, and they would kill you in a second if they knew you had that kind of cash on you."

"Thanks, Alex. All is good on my end. I will see you in a month."

They left each other, Kenny continuing south, encircling the zoo, looking like any other walker in the park enjoying a nice summer day. He headed out of the park on Tamm Avenue towards Dogtown, the truest Irish neighborhood in St. Louis, for lunch and a beer at Seamus Mc-Daniel's. He cradled the backpack, knowing that at least $50,000 of the $200,000 would be his at month's end. While he knew he had to pay commissions to at least 10 of his guys, he assumed a few would not be alive at the end of the month to receive theirs, so he would add their take to his. That is what Kenny loved about Alex's latest scam. Alex did not care where the money went and wanted no paper or electronic trail. The revenue generated from the insurance policies was of no concern to Alex. His payout came after the policy's death benefit was paid off, and unlike any other insurance company on earth, they wanted to pay out the death benefit. Unlike other insurance policies that were more profitable, if the policy lasted years and years, Alex profited if the death benefit paid off quickly. Alex would make nearly 30 times the value of the policy's death benefit. Kenny laughed to himself as he found a chair at the bar. He knew that all he had to do was line them up and let society knock them down. That statement was sort of the unwritten mission statement of the TTWC Insurance Company.

Alex walked east towards The Center, and not having a backpack with $200,000 made his steps lighter, but it was not due to the missing weight. It was from his feeling that he could control life and death. Alex was such a narcissist that he felt all his actions, ideas, and plans were his way of improving society. In his warped mind, he contemplated that he would be listed in history books not only as one of the most innovative entrepreneurs in history but a leader in medical breakthroughs and societal transformation. It did not matter to him that thousands of families, unbeknownst to them, would just be raw materials in the supply and demand chain of organs.

CHAPTER 32

❧

Vinnie had spent the entire evening researching all he could on transplants. He studied trends nationally and locally by race, income, gender, and type of transplant needed. He also studied Frank's disease in-depth, and after hours in front of his computer, his eyes raw and red from reading and his spirits drained, he reached two conclusions. First, Frank was screwed unless he got a transplant soon. Secondly, Vinnie could not just let this fall to fate. The problem seemed overwhelming, and he appeared paralyzed as to what his first move should be. He felt he had to do something about it, but where to start was his dilemma.

Although it was nearly 9:00 p.m., he reached out to the one person over the last 35 years who could also help sort things out for him. *Damn it*, he thought, *why do I still need her?* As he texted: "Ellen, need to talk with you tomorrow. Important. Please call when able."

Instantly, his phone pinged a return message from Ellen saying: "Come over tomorrow morning to my place for breakfast. 7:00 a.m. too early?"

He wrote back: "Not too early. See you there." Then adding, for a reason he did not know, "Have a good night."

He was too exhausted to relive past wars with Ellen, but going to her place, which only a few years ago was their place, still touched a nerve with him. When they were together, Ellen contributed much more to their household income. So, their home, a luxury condo in the Chase Park Plaza Building with the best view in the city overlooking Forest Park, was picked out by her. Primarily because of its proximity to the hospital complex. She also decorated it to satisfy her love for entertainment; a chore Vinnie preferred to avoid and one of the reasons they divorced. In the settlement, Ellen generously paid Vinnie more than 50% of the condo's value so she could stay there. In the divorce, neither Ellen nor Vinnie treated the other unkindly, and their significant financial assets, in most cases, were divided equally, if not benefiting Vinnie. While Vinnie appreciated the fairness of Ellen in the divorce, he still had a chip on his shoulder, and while it should be getting smaller, it was getting bigger due to her success and ability to move on, something he seemed not to be able to do. With his focus on Frank, though, he began realizing some things in life like money and possessions did not matter. People you loved mattered. Being a better person mattered. Helping those in need mattered. To turn off the Ellen switch for the night, he went to his bedroom and turned on the TV, catching the last few innings of the Cardinal game. Seeing they were losing again by seven runs to the first-place Milwaukee Brewers, he said, laughing to himself and turning off the lights, *"Know what else matters? Goddamn starting pitching and clutch hitting."*

The following day Vinnie was well-rested and of a clear conscience as he headed off to Ellen's condo, which was only a few miles away on Kingshighway. Vinnie was never very considerate when visiting people in their homes when he and Ellen were married. However, he did stop at Panera Bread, originally the St. Louis Bread Company and still referred to locally as BreadCo., to pick up a couple of Bear Claw pastries. He knew no matter how much Ellen may be dieting, although she never needed to, she would graciously accept and enjoy the pastry. Parking in Ellen's guest spot, Vinnie walked into the residence lobby and was met by the doorman, Ernie, a bear of a man, an old friend, and a reminder of a life Vinnie lived before the divorce.

"Well, look who the cat dragged in," Ernie bellowed as he put his massive arms around Vinnie. "I never thought I would see you crawling back to Dr. Calabrese's doorstep."

"Well, for a long time, it was my doorstep, too, Ernie. Besides, I think I left a bottle of scotch here two years ago, and I have come to retrieve it, my good man. And if it weren't 7:00 in the morning, I would share a nip with you on the way out."

"If you don't come out in an hour, I will come to rescue you and that bottle of scotch, but don't be confused. It's the scotch I am trying to save, not you."

Ernie laughed as he dialed the phone to Ellen's apartment. "Dr. Calabrese, good morning. I have a straggly-looking gentleman that claims to be your ex-husband. May I send him up?"

Vinnie stood in silence as Ernie laughed at something Ellen said. Ernie hung up the phone and said, "The Doctor will see you, sir."

"What was so funny, Ernie?"

"Well, Dr. Calabrese wanted to make sure that if you were not out of there in an hour, I would come up and rescue her. I guess the more things change, the more they stay the same, right, Vinnie? Let me get that elevator for you."

Ernie patted Vinnie on the back, stepped in the elevator to press 20, and then stepped out saying, as the doors closed, "Don't forget the scotch, Vinnie."

Riding up the elevator to the 20th floor, Vinnie silently thought about his life when he lived here. How many late nights did he share a sip of whisky and a little two-way advice with Ernie as he grabbed a smoke outside? While Vinnie tried to convince himself he was happy, there was so much of the past life he missed. While certainly not a loner, it seemed to him he was more and more alone. He told himself that his loneliness was not why his encounters with Ellen had increased over the last several months. This visit had the purpose of helping Frank, and with that, Vinnie knocked on the door.

Ellen answered, "Impeccably dressed, as always, even if it was 7:00 in the morning." To Vinnie's surprise, Ellen kissed him on the cheek when he entered. Seeing the look of surprise on Vinnie's face, Ellen simply shrugged and said, "Old habits."

"Speaking of old habits, I assume you still like these?" Vinnie asked as he handed Ellen the Panera bag with the Bear Claws. Looking inside, she shook her head and smiled. "Old and bad habits, but thank you. I am glad I have not eaten, so I have no excuse not to enjoy these."

They walked to the kitchen table that Ellen had set out with an assortment of juices, coffee, and cereals. Ellen added the Bear Claws to the plates and offered Vinnie a chair with a panoramic view of the park.

"Boy, I do miss this view," Vinnie said as he looked out the window. From the 20th floor, all the features of the entire park seemed within reach. The park had always been Vinnie's place of solitude and thinking, and he still visited it three to four times a week.

"You know, Vinnie, every once in a while, I look out on Jefferson Lake, and I think I've seen you fishing," Ellen said.

"Well, you might have caught me looking up at you if you have. Though sometimes it is hard remembering where your windows are in the building. My eyesight is not as good as it used to be."

Sensing an uncomfortable pause in the conversation and wanting to move it past old memories or avoid making new ones, Ellen curtly said, "Vinnie, you said you needed to talk, and you sounded as if it was urgent. What's up?"

Ellen poured herself and Vinnie coffee, and they both took a Bear Claw. After a bite of the pastry and a sip of coffee, Vinnie explained why he needed to talk to Ellen.

"How aware are you of Frank's situation with his lungs?" Vinnie asked.

"Well, in talking to you and our girls, who talk to Frank and Sue's kids, I think I am up to speed on him, but I have not gotten an update in almost a month. Why has something significantly changed?"

"I am not sure. I think Frank is going downhill fast."

"Why do you say that? In what way is he going downhill?" Ellen asked.

"He has such difficulty breathing. His movements are incredibly labored, and while he is trying to lose weight and get healthy to be eligible for a transplant, I think he may run out of time."

Solemnly Ellen stared at Vinnie and simply said, "Unfortunately, with patients like Frank, time is never on their side."

"That's why I am here, Ellen. Can you do something to help him?"

"Like what?" Ellen asked.

"Can you find him a lung, get him to the front of the line like those rich assholes seem to be able to do? Is that possible, Ellen?" Vinnie said while wringing his hands and looking down as he said it.

Sensing Vinnie's despair, Ellen got up instinctively and walked around the table to put her arm around him. Kneeling to be at eye level with him, she said, "I am sorry, Vinnie, there is nothing I can do for him. The Center currently must work within the confines of the transplant process. Frank's turn will come when and if Frank's turn comes, and he is doing the right thing by working very hard to get in better health."

Staring back at Ellen, his eyes misty with tears but glowing red and turning to anger, Vinnie lashed out at Ellen.

"That's cold, Ellen. His turn will come when or if it comes. What bullshit is that? Is that how you comfort your patients?"

Without rising anger in her voice, Ellen said, "As a matter of fact, yes, that is what I tell my patients. There is no guarantee any of them will ever get a transplant, and they need to understand the realities of what they will be dealing with. Running out of time, never having a match, or having an organ rejected. It's a crap shoot, Vinnie, and the odds for Frank are bad."

"But I thought The Center was doing breakthrough things in transplants. Right? That is what you told me."

"Yes, we are, but it is still a supply and demand business, and until we get more people willing to donate, we won't be able to supply those organs for all those who need them. We are working on that, but it's a long haul, too long, unfortunately, for Frank. He needs lungs in weeks or months, and The Center won't be of much help in the short term. The only thing I can do, Vinnie, and I will gladly do it, is to look at Frank's medical situation and talk to his pulmonologist. I can ensure Frank and his doctors are doing everything to increase his odds of getting a match, but I am sure he and his doctors are covering all of that."

Glumly, Vinnie sat up and said, "Well, I guess the great Alex Finnegan does not walk on water after all. I would think that anyone with his size ego would be able to snap his fingers and get what we need with ease."

Knowing that mention of Alex triggered anger in Vinnie, Ellen decided there was nothing more that could come out of this conversation, so she tried to console Vinnie a bit. "Vinnie, let me investigate and maybe talk to Alex to see if he has any ideas, but don't hold out hope and don't share any of this with Frank. I do not want him veering from the plan he and his doctors have laid out. Encourage him to work hard to get in shape and get healthier."

As he got up to leave, Vinnie hugged Ellen, perhaps longer than she felt comfortable, but neither pulled away. "Ellen, one last favor. Do you have a bottle of scotch I can take with me?"

Ellen grabbed a bottle of Glenlivet from the bar and handed it to Vinnie. As she ushered him to the door, she said, "Say hi to Ernie for me. I think a conversation with him could help you right now."

As Vinnie left, Ellen wondered why she had just lied to Vinnie. She knew that if they wanted to, Alex and herself could break the rules as that is what she and Alex had just discussed after the investor meeting. The whole basis of The Center's success was to break the rules, to push the envelope. The question was, would she or Alex do it for Vinnie and Frank?

CHAPTER 33

Rhonda and Angie Sullivan met as planned on Friday at Angie's office at 4:00 p.m. While the two street-hardened vets rarely showed a soft side to their colleagues, they greeted each other with warm hugs to rekindle their friendship and feel the kinship of being females in a dangerous job male-oriented culture. Screw what other cops thought of their friendship. They knew too well that their colleagues and good friends were no longer alive, working in the hell they worked in, and they would cherish any chance to reconnect as humans.

"Rhonda, we are all set up in the conference room to watch the videos you had me procure. But before we do, what were you saying about buying dinner if you find a white Audi on one of the videos?"

Knowing Angie never asked a question she did not know the answer to, she assumed Angie had already scoured the videos and spotted the Audi to ensure a free dinner. Rhonda sat down in the conference room and jokingly said, "So, Sully," her nickname for Angie, "do you just want to fast forward to the Audi, or do you want to go through the motions of looking at all the videos?"

"Hell, Rhonda, I am too busy to do your work for you. Just look at the damn videos. All of them." Then laughing, "But hurry. We have 6:30 reservations for dinner."

Rhonda started the first security video, showing the parking garage of McConnell and McGrath corporate law offices. The attempted carjacking and murder occurred around 8:30 p.m. when McConnell and McGrath's lawyer, Kim DeAngelo, was leaving work from her 10th-floor office. Working long hours to earn the coveted partner status at the firm was not uncommon for Ms. DeAngelo. Based on interviews after the crime was committed, her friends and associates told the police they always cautioned Kim to arrive and leave in daylight hours. Some recommended she carry a gun as downtown St. Louis, in their opinion, was not safe. From her perspective, downtown was safe if you knew your surroundings. As far as carrying a gun, never. As she told friends often, she hoped she would live her entire life never so afraid that having a gun would give her a false sense of security. Kim DeAngelo always believed in the goodness of people, and maybe, her naivety got her killed.

Rhonda reviewed the video of the garage at the time the crime occurred. She saw Ms. DeAngelo leaving the 3rd-floor garage elevator and walking to her car. She was aware of her surroundings and doing what safety guidelines instructed people, especially women, to do. Walk briskly and confidently, hold your keys in your hands, keep your valuables such as briefcases or purses close to your body, and keep your eyes alert for any impending danger.

Rhonda then turned to the footage of the cameras pointing at the stairwell entrances. As Ms. DeAngelo walked to her car, Rhonda saw two black males appear from the stairwell and begin making their way toward Ms. DeAngelo. Going back to the footage that shows the larger garage area and Ms. DeAngelo walking to her car, Rhonda could tell by her motions that she was aware of the two males approaching. However, Rhonda soon saw the real threat that, unfortunately, Ms. DeAngelo did not. Another male approached her car from the opposite side of the garage. It was obvious to Rhonda that all three were working together as the two males exiting the staircase were too far to assault Ms. DeAngelo before she reached her car, perhaps giving her a false sense of security. However, the lone male was within feet of Ms. DeAngelo. With her eyes looking left, Ms. DeAngelo got blindsided by the blow to her head from her right. As Ms. DeAngelo went down in a heap, the other two males raced towards the car and grabbed her keys, purse, and briefcase. They started her car and quickly accelerated out of the garage, or so they thought. Soon it was apparent based on the starts and stops of the vehicle, a newer model Porsche 911, that they were having trouble driving the car. It was a manual stick shift. The cameras then showed the two men leaving the vehicle and running back towards the exit. The solitary man did not run but stared down at Ms. DeAngelo, still lying on the pavement from the initial blow to her head. He calmly took out a handgun and shot her twice, at point-blank range.

Perhaps he wanted no witnesses, or his job was not finished until Ms. DeAngelo was dead. Or maybe, he was pissed off that the car was a stick shift. Regardless of how often Detective Simon had seen crimes on video, it sickened her of the hatred one human being could have towards another. However, as bad as the footage of the actual crime was, this was not the footage she was most interested in.

She turned to Angie, saying, "Before we compare footage of your three assailants to the footage of my cop haters who wished me well after the Thomson murder, let's go back an hour before they committed the crime and 15 minutes after these three assholes left the garage."

"Ok, Rhonda," Angie said as she set up the playback for the street cameras, "do you think we are looking at the same guys?"

"Crimes committed less than a mile from each other. About the same time of night. Victim walking alone, or in Mr. Thomson's case, with a non-threatening associate, his grandson. Yep. I would bet they are the same guys. What I want to know, though, is if the white Audi is in play here?"

Soon Detectives Sullivan and Simon would have one answer, but it would open many more questions. They sat and reviewed street cameras from 8th and 9th streets, east and west of the parking garage, and north and south on Olive and Locust Streets. Any place the assailants could leave the garage would be seen with these cameras. Rhonda went back in 15-minute increments, and a camera with footage from 8th street clearly showed the three assailants entering the garage on the ground floor; the floor on which Ms. DeAngelo was carjacked was three floors up. She went back another 15 minutes, then 30 minutes, to see if the white Audi had appeared with the three men before the crime occurred as it had with the carjacking after the ball game. Nothing. It seemed the assailants had walked to the law office location, or if they did get dropped off, it was in an area that these cameras did not cover. There were hundreds of cameras within a three or four-block area of the building, and unless she had a firm connection of the Audi to the crimes, she would not be able to request the resources to review all the possible footage.

She then decided to look at footage from the street cameras immediately after the crime. While she did pick up the assailants leaving from the same garage entrance as they had entered, she did not see them make any contact with the Audi or any car for that matter. She noticed how the three men coolly walked out of the garage as if they had parked their car and then headed off on a stroll downtown. There was no panic in their gait or expressions as they were laughing. One of the men took out his cell phone, put it to his ear, and had a quick conversation with someone. Placing the cell in his pants pocket, he motioned the other two, indicating a change in direction, and instead of continuing south on 8th street, they took a quick left and headed east on Olive towards the Gateway Arch. About 100 feet after they turned east on Olive, Rhonda noticed a white Audi drive by them on Olive, but it did not stop, slow down, nor did the three assailants look up to show any sign of recognition or expectation. The Audi drove on, but Detective Simon could pick up a Missouri plate reading: TTWC 21.

Pausing to think, she turned off the video and turned to Angie Sullivan.

"What do you think, Sully? Is there a connection between this Audi and the carjackers?"

"Well, if you think it is connected, you can convince me over the dinner you are buying."

Rhonda shook her head and said, "I think I need a drink more than food after watching that shitshow."

They left the precinct in separate cars as they would go in different directions home after dinner. Settling in a darkened back booth at McGurk's, one of their favorite eating and drinking spots, they quickly motioned the waiter over, and each ordered a glass of Jameson's Irish Whisky neat.

Clinking their glasses together, they offered their traditional toast: "Here's to the good guys, and may the bad ones rot in hell." They quickly took a long sip of the whisky, finishing the healthy pour quickly. After a hard day, the whiskey had an immediate calming effect, like taking a deep breath or inhaling the first drag on a cigarette though neither detective smoked. They signaled for another round, but the waiter was one step ahead, already walking over with two more drinks in his hands as he knew they were cops, and he knew the pace cops kept when they let off steam after work.

They sipped the second round more slowly and looked at the menu. While both knew they would get completely shit-faced, they still had to review what they just saw while sober, giving them about 30 more minutes of clarity.

Rhonda asked, "So what do you think we got?"

Angie summarized while sipping her whisky. "I know we got three assholes, killing an innocent woman for kicks, money, street cred, or whatever the hell motivates them. That I know, we got. Now, we likely have the same little darlings doing the same rite of passage at your crime scene. I want to emphasize likely. I don't know till we compare my footage with yours, which I will do tomorrow as soon as my guaranteed hangover from tonight clears up. And finally, what we may have or hope to have is a connection with the two crime scenes and your white Audi. But that is a big maybe."

"And, my dear Angie," Rhonda said while patting Angie's hand, "we do have a plate for the Audi." Rhonda looked at her notes and said, "Let's not forget Mr. TTWC 21."

"Maybe, Rhonda. Lots of Audi's in St. Louis. Trendy car, extremely common color as well. But it is easily checked out. Why don't you run the plates on the car, and I will spend time comparing videos and checking our other carjacking cases to see if anything else connects with these two events."

They both took a minute to peruse the menu once more, and then the waiter took their identical order: Cheeseburgers, medium rare, the works on top, and fries on the side. Rhonda said to the waiter as she handed back the menus, "If the streets don't kill us, the dinner table will."

Their laughter subsided as two ice-cold Budweiser bottles landed on their table.

In between sips of the beer, Angie asked, "Rhonda, how do you think the Audi may be involved? You know it's pretty much: See, Take, Run, and occasionally Kill. Few carjackers get private transportation to do the jacking or call an uber. Usually, not a lot of long-term planning goes into these things."

Rhonda answered her with more questions. "What if the driver of the Audi is more interested in securing the car after it stealing it? Maybe that's their interest. Many carjackers do it for a quick score and leave the car a few miles away."

Angie answered, "Maybe, but the Audi driver does not have to be nearby to ensure they receive the stolen car. He could have the carjackers leave it a few miles from the crime scene. Much easier. It seems like they are taking a lot of risks staying close. They know there is a damn camera on every street corner as well as we do. Is there any connection between Kim DeAngelo and Bill Thomson besides the possible white Audi and the assailants?"

"Hmm, seems like a long shot but probably has to be checked out," Rhonda answered. "But if I am checking that out, I need to check out the possible connection with William Burroughs's killing, but that seems like a real long shot."

"William Burroughs?" Angie asked in a confused tone. "The north side drug dealer whose second home has been Potosi Correctional every other year for the last ten years?"

"Well, he has a new home now. Much warmer in the winter," Rhonda answered.

"Did he move down south?" Angie asked quizzically.

"Sort of. He is in hell. He is dead. Happened a few weeks back," said Rhonda adding, "He was number 89 on our city murder 2021 countdown."

"Wow, I need to keep up on things. I am focused 24/7 on these carjackings and guess not keeping up with the overall murder scene. What are we up to now?"

"97," replied Rhonda, "but I am betting on a long hot summer to get us well on our way over 200 for the year. And since the news about William Burroughs has got your attention, Angie, how about this? One of the few tips we got was a white Audi was seen dropping off two males at the house where Burroughs was killed 20 minutes later."

Angie thought aloud, "Three murders, questionable if connected because the victims don't seem to have anything in common. Both the crimes were downtown, but those areas are distinctly different neighborhoods. One is a business district that empties after 6:00 p.m., and one, the ballpark area, comes to life after 6:00. Plus, Burroughs is killed in north city 15 miles away with no jacking involved. It seems the only constant of the three crimes is maybe the white Audi, but we are not even sure it is the same car. Now, if you can connect the carjacking perps to William Burroughs's crime scene and the white Audi to all or at least two of the three scenes, then we may have something, my dear Detective Simon."

"Well, I can't do that yet, Sully, but you have earned your dinner tonight. We have a lot of work tomorrow, but let's have one last drink before I pay. You have been a great help and a great friend. I needed this night to work through some things but, more importantly, help take the edge off this crap job of mine - at least for a few hours."

Hugging once more as they left the restaurant and headed toward their cars, Sully whispered to Rhonda, "Go get those bad guys and send them to hell."

CHAPTER 34

❧✦❧

While unsure but suspecting Alex's intentions, Brooke turned down his invitation for dinner on Saturday night, sensing it sounded more like a date. She agreed to meet him on Thursday night at SqWires Restaurant in Lafayette Square, where she lived and a few miles south of the hospital complex. At nearly 200 years old, Lafayette Square was one of the oldest areas in St. Louis and featured stately Victorian homes from the mid-1800s, surrounding Lafayette Park, the city's first park. St. Louis comprises many neighborhoods, each depicting the European influence of those who first settled in the area. The heavy German influence was impacted by the great beer barons who settled in St. Louis in the mid-1800s. The Italian area, the Hill, featured an abundance of great restaurants strewn throughout a neighborhood of neatly maintained, small brick homes passed down by generations from the families of the immigrants who arrived in the early 1900s. The French areas consist of Lafayette Square and the adjacent Soulard area, home to the second-largest Mardi Gras celebration after New Orleans. The French areas were the oldest in St. Louis and extensions of the first French settlers from the late 1700s.

It was these areas, and especially Lafayette Square that Brooke liked best. She leased a two-bedroom apartment that was originally a carriage house behind a Victorian mansion on Park and Mississippi Ave, a short walk to the restaurant. The restaurant was staffed with friends of hers, and while she could certainly handle herself, it was nice to be able to signal to her friends for help. Brooke liked controlling her environment when it was unknown, and what she was walking into with Alex Finnegan was still unknown. On several dates gone bad, she had employed this tactic but could not believe someone as accomplished as Alex Finnegan would turn into a handsy jerk like so many of the younger men she dated. But as she always reminded herself, young or old, rich or poor, all men could act like jerks if not properly managed.

Arriving at the restaurant 30 minutes early to chat with her friends and pick out a good table, she surfed the web on her phone, reading up on the latest info on Alex Finnegan. There was plenty of news about him and Arch City Transplant. Most of this information Brooke had already researched and had known. What she was searching for was more information on his private life. Brooke assumed he was single, but he would not be the first married man to forget he was married while pursuing her. She was unsure, and after a few keywords typed into Google, she found herself immersed in the personal side of Dr. Finnegan. Beyond running and working, it seemed his other interests were attending numerous charity functions in town, depicted in photos featuring him, and what it appeared, a different beautiful woman beaming by his side. Perhaps she wondered, Alex changed out women for events like women changed out shoes.

While studying the personal life of Alex Finnegan, Brooke heard a voice behind her saying, "That guy looks like a real asshole."

Before turning to see who was speaking, she laughed and said, "He probably is. Most men I meet are."

"Well, you will find out tonight as he is your dinner companion," Alex laughed as he tapped her on the shoulder, and she turned towards him, knowing she had put her foot in her mouth but did not care as she thought it best that Alex Finnegan did not get the upper hand tonight.

"I guess that was a good ice breaker for the evening," Brooke said. Alex replied, "Well, most of the women I date think the same thing but usually after the date, not before."

"Ok, but let's start over and call this a business meeting rather than a date. Agreed, Dr. Finnegan?"

"So, it is. Let's get a table and get down to business, Brooke."

They walked to a nearby table that Brooke had picked out, which gave a full floor-length view of SqWire's unique atmosphere. It was an early 19th-century wire factory, still displaying pully systems, industrial ceiling fans, and fireplaces, transformed into a modern farm-to-table restaurant. There were over 40 of these types of renovated restaurants occupying the buildings that remained from the era of Victorian splendor in St. Louis.

Passing on ordering a cocktail and choosing to order sparkling water, Brooke wanted to set the tone immediately that this was not a social dinner. Surprisingly, Alex had the same, saying he had another appointment after dinner and had an early day tomorrow. That was the first surprise Brooke would get from Dr. Finnegan tonight, but it would not be the last.

"Brooke, why don't you order some appetizers so we can talk while we eat? Besides, my next meeting is also at a restaurant, and I don't want to fill up here, as I am sure I will have to eat later. Despite all the running I do, work appointments at restaurants do add the pounds on," Alex said as he patted, what Brooke assumed, was his ripped abs.

While Brooke ordered from Brian, the waiter, and one of her good friends, Alex got down to business as promised.

"Brooke, it is not for social reasons that Ellen and I have met with you so many times and each time seemed like we were interrogating you. The simple truth is we both want and need you to become part of our team at Arch City Transplant Center. We are building something that will change people's lives, and it will change your life if you join us."

While not surprised that a job was in the offering, as Brooke suspected she was interviewing, she was surprised by what came next.

"You would be the Director of Transplantation Synergy, and we will double your current salary. And we will provide you, as we do with all key employees, stock options that when we go public could make you a millionaire at a very young age."

Brooke's head was spinning, and she was glad she had not ordered a drink but knew she would need one once this dinner was over.

"I am flattered, Dr. Finnegan, and do appreciate all the time you and Dr. Calabrese have spent with me, but this seems so sudden and unexpected. I love what I am doing at the hospital, and it seems I am getting my footing there. I am not sure I am ready to take on a job that it seems, based on the compensation you are offering me, more than I am ready for."

"Brooke, we studied you, your education, and your work history. We know you are an overachiever, a fast learner, and both compassionate and a risk-taker. We also know you will outgrow your job in a few years and while you can continue to excel and prosper to a comfortable level at the hospital, what we are offering you goes beyond comfort. We are offering you the chance to be part of the transformational change we are making in health care, science, transplantations, and our society. You will not only be saving lives but also changing lives, including yours."

"Can you be more specific? The title, what was it? Director of Transplantation Synergy sounds a little nebulous. What does that mean?" Brooke asked.

"I can give you a broad overview of what the job entails, but much of the inner workings of The Center's operations and your role in it will be unveiled to you after you agree to our offer and come on board. But, we don't want to provide confidential information to a job candidate unless we know they will join us."

"That makes sense, Dr. Finnegan. When we were together, you gave me a pretty broad overview of what The Center hopes to achieve and change, but you were about to discuss a major change or shift in thinking about transplants that The Center would also need to address, but you got a phone call, and we never got to that."

"You're right, and that piece of it is a key part of your job that I hope we have time to discuss tonight." Then looking at his watch, Dr. Finnegan said, "So let me dive in before I need to run to my next appointment."

"What we are doing, what you will be doing, is upending the current thinking on the handling of transplants, and I think after your tour and our past conversations, you got a general sense of what that is. As you already know, some of our thinking threatens the current system, including your present employer. However, to make our vision come true, we need to change the donor supply chain, which requires a shift in how society views transplants. That shift will not occur with posters at the doctor's offices and the DMV to encourage becoming a donor. It will occur by changing the stakes and fortunes of those who become donors."

"What shifts are you talking about, and how will you create that change?" Brooke interrupted.

"Well, most people think the way to enact change, or in this case, laws involving transplants is through the legislative process in Washington. But since it has been about 40 years since Washington implemented any major legislation on transplants, I am not holding my breath that we can rely on laws, in my lifetime, to change the process."

"I would agree with you, Dr. Finnegan. So, how do you speed up the process?" Brooke asked.

"Well, in a young person's vocabulary, we take it to the streets. We create a movement from the ground up, voiced by people, forcing our politicians to act, and if they don't act, which they won't in the time frame The Center needs, we take matters into our own hands and push against accepted norms, even accepted laws. When we are successful, not if, we will have money and political clout to get the laws changed to favor our concept."

"That sounds very big picture, but I am still unclear about my role in all of this," Brooke asked.

"Like any movement, there are those unseen, working the back channels, greasing the wheels with politicians, influencers, and investors. That is my role. Your role is to be our customer-facing individual, explaining and selling our concept to the people who would benefit from these changes we seek."

Brooke said nothing, so Finnegan continued.

"You would be our public-facing executive, convincing donors and recipients that our process is the best process in which they can participate. You would be with them on every step they take on the transplant journey. You would handle bringing our message to larger groups who have considerable sway over the decisions donors and recipient families need to make. By talking to clergy, doctors assisted living facilities, and family members, you will hopefully convince those who have not agreed to become a donor to do so. You will convince those agreeing to donate to do so through The Center versus going through the current process."

"But the current process works, Dr. Finnegan."

"The current processes administered by the government and implemented by hospitals, which, while mostly for profit, are not, in my opinion, run like a privatized business. Too many regulations, and thus they are restrained or stay within the lines. The Transplant Center is privatizing transplants and will do so by making money by securing donors and securing recipients in a non-traditional, entrepreneurial, capitalistic way."

"How will you do that?" Brooke asked.

"By giving people options that today they don't have. That is the difference between capitalism and communism. Choice. Today, as a donor, you do not have a choice. Today as a recipient, you do not have a choice. You are a number in a database that relies on the right person dying at the right time, and if you are lucky, your number gets called. Brooke, you have seen first-hand how random this process is. That is why we want you to join us so much. You have seen good families get passed by on organs because of a matching formula. You know our demand greatly outstrips our supply. And just wait till the long-term effects of Covid hit the lung transplant supply and demand chain. More people will die because there is no supply, and the demand, especially for lungs, will increase ten-fold."

"Doctor, I am realistic about working within our system, and I certainly know it has issues, but what you are talking about seems to be upending how the entire medical industry handles transplants."

"I, and hopefully you, if you join us, will be a disrupter. No different than any business that created a better way than in the past. iPhones, Uber, PayPal, Netflix, Amazon, Stripe, Crypto-currency, telemedicine. The list goes on and on of companies or services that did not exist ten years ago but are now part of our everyday lives. Why should medicine and transplants be immune from disruptive change? You know, Brooke, no law says that when someone agrees to donate an organ, they must go through with it. It still requires the family's consent. No law says a donor's family can't know who the donor is. And while there is a national consensus on the right to die, eight states allow physician-assisted suicide for terminal patients. Why not allow those who want to be donors also to choose when and how they want to die? You hear this phrase all the time with the abortion debate, and now Covid with masks and vaccines. "My body, my rights, my decision."

"Yes, I have heard the phrase, and I know everyone uses it to their advantage based on what side of the debate they are on," Brooke said calmly and introspectively.

"That phase and the politicization of that phase is what we will hang our vision on. People on both sides use that phase to keep the government out of our lives. It has always been a rallying cry for abortion rights, and now Covid shutdowns, vaccines, and mask mandates, but I believe it will become a rallying cry for how we choose to die and what we choose to do with our organs when we die."

Brooke's head was spinning.

"Brooke, if you believe as I do, the government has no place in telling us what we can do with our bodies, then you have to believe the ultimate ownership of that right begins with how we choose to die and when we do, how we choose to donate or not donate our organs. While physician-assisted suicide is only one piece of my strategy for The Center because we can greatly improve donor supply without it, I am willing and driven to knock that cultural stigma down as well. Polls have shown that the public, left and right is more accepting than ever of some form of physician-assisted suicide. So, momentum and legal decisions siding with the patient will eventually make this more commonplace, and when it is, the Transplant Center will benefit. All I am saying, Brooke, is giving your organs is the ultimate sacrifice one can make, the gift of their body, their life, so shouldn't everything surrounding it be solely a personal decision?"

Brooke just sat quietly, processing all that Dr. Finnegan had said. He sat there, quietly but confidently, feeling he had her on his side. Finally, Brooke spoke, "I can tell you, Dr. Finnegan, every meeting or conversation I have with you and Dr. Calabrese has both excited me and, to be honest with you, scared me a little bit. I cannot commit yet, but you have my attention."

"Well, good. Hopefully, this dinner will end with you not thinking I am an asshole though you may think that after working with me. I know I have thrown a lot at you, and you should consider it. Talk to Ellen or me again. I would ask, though, that you do not talk to anyone at the hospital about our conversation as that is probably not good for us or you at this stage."

Alex paid the check and then got up from the table, patting Brooke lightly on her knee. "Brooke, I am sorry to cut this meeting short, but I have another appointment. Please get back to Ellen or me on whatever questions you have." Alex left, and Brooke's friend Brian came by on cue to check up on her. "That was quick. Did everything go ok, Brooke?"

"Yeah, Brian. I think so, but meet me at the bar and grab me a vodka on the rocks. I could use a sounding board. My life may have just taken a major turn."

CHAPTER 35

Alex did not have far to go for his next meeting, as its location was planned in conjunction with the dinner with Brooke. He hopped in his car and drove a mile north to a restaurant called Vin de Set. It had a great rooftop view of the city. Alex took the stairs up three floors to its location and settled in a booth across from Ellen as she asked him about the evening's developments.

"Based on the look on your face, you seem pleased with how the conversation went with Brooke."

"You know, Ellen, I consider myself a closer, whether I am chasing women or closing business deals, and while she has some thinking she wants to do, I would say we will get her on our team," Alex boasted.

"Let's focus on closing her for our business and not for your bed, Alex. We have too much riding on this and her for you to put your libido above our bottom line. Besides, Alex, every time I pull up the society pages in the Ladue News, I see you with yet another beauty on your arm. I think you can leave Brooke out of your trophy room."

"Fine. I will behave," Alex said, but in a way in which Ellen knew he was placating her. Alex chased women like he chased business deals: to win at all costs.

Ellen wanted to move past Brooke and discuss with Alex another subject she had been thinking of since she last met Vinnie. She never wanted Alex to feel that he owed her a favor as she never wanted Alex to have any more leverage than he currently had with her, but she did need Alex's help.

"Alex, I will get back to Brooke in a few days, but let's change the subject as I want to run something else by you."

"Ok, shoot, Ellen. What is it that I can do for you?"

"Well, maybe nothing more than giving me your opinion because I know anything more will result in payback from me to you, but I need your thinking around a case involving my former brother-in-law. His name is Frank Esposito, and he is on the waiting list for a double lung transplant. He has Interstitial Fibrosis and has been working on getting himself into better shape to be eligible for a transplant when he can accept one."

"That's a horrible illness. The problem is, Frank, is running out of time, right, Ellen?" Alex responded matter-of-factly, as he had seen this scenario play out so many times.

"Yes, he is running out of time, and Vinnie came by to see me the other morning. I have never seen him so emotionally on edge. He asked me if there was anything I could do to help Frank, and of course, playing by the book, I told him there was nothing I could do."

"You're right, Ellen. There is nothing you can do, so why are you asking me?"

"Because Alex, you don't play by the book. You love rewriting the book or ignoring the pages you disagree with as long as it achieves your goals."

"Guilty, but while I have sympathy for your brother-in-law, why the hell should I do something for your ex-husband. No offense, Ellen, but he is an asshole."

"I hope that despite whatever grudges you and Vinnie have, you would at least consider doing this favor for me."

"Quid pro quo, Ellen. What will you do for me if I help you out here?"

"Yeah, and Vinnie is the asshole," Ellen laughed. "You just can't see the benefit of helping someone unless you get some sort of payback, can you, Alex?"

"Nope. If I see no advantage, then why waste my time helping people who cannot benefit me?"

"I'm curious, Alex. How does Kenny Thorton benefit you as you seem to help him quite a bit? It seems to me for a guy who has not worked consistently for the last five years, who probably still has a pretty good monthly drug and booze tab, he certainly lives a nice life, thanks to you."

"Kenny is a lifelong good friend, and I give him some projects from time to time. He has had a tough life, and I don't want him to end back up in prison."

Sensing she had hit a nerve, Ellen decided to apply pressure on Alex. She knew she was one of the few people in Alex's life who could apply pressure.

"You know, Alex, you can't lie and try to charm the pants off me like you think you can with Brooke or any other woman you seduce. I know too much about you, and what I know about you is while you are brilliant, you need someone to do your dirty work for you, and Kenny, I guess that someone. Probably been your entire life, and that is how he helps you. Either that, or he has something on you."

Alex shifted in his seat, a nervous tell Ellen always looked for when pressing Alex.

"Are you done, Ellen? God, you are such a ballbuster," Alex said with a smile. "That is why I put up with you and your bullshit because you and I want the same things in life. And while we might pursue them in different ways, the goal is the same. Win at all costs. Right, Ellen?"

Ellen sat wistfully, knowing that Alex was probably right and her win at all costs approach probably was a factor in her failed marriage to Vinnie, but in her mind, there were lines that Alex would cross that she would not. Letting her silence push Alex to make the next move, another trait of his she played perfectly, Alex finally responded.

"Ok, get me the information on your brother-in-law, but just deliver it to me verbally. I don't want his medical records in your hands or mine. Get any details you can from him directly or, if need be, try and access his pulmonologist records but avoid any written or electronic communications as much as possible. Also, don't give your ex-husband any updates beyond general ones. I don't need to run into him at the club and have him ask me questions. He is a bit of a violent loose wire."

Ellen knew everything Alex asked her to do she had already thought of, and they were safe standard requests. She knew she could talk to Frank's pulmonologist, as well, without raising any eyebrows. She might even know him. She was concerned about how off the books Alex wanted the information. She suspected that any solution Alex came up with would not be written up in the medical journals, and she was hoping it wouldn't show up in police journals, either. She also understood his desire to keep Vinnie in the dark as Vinnie had a big chip on his shoulder regarding Alex, and she did not need to have that drama enter this delicate situation.

"Alex, I want to make sure you are not planning to do anything illegal. I am not asking you for that. Let me be clear on that."

"I am not going to do anything but look at his records to see what path we may be able to take. And no offense, Ellen, but I would not jeopardize our business and future for your ex-brother-in-law. Sorry, but we have more lives to save than just his." Warily looking into his eyes, believing that she had possibly made a deal with the devil, she nonetheless thanked him for looking into the case.

"Oh, and one last thing, Ellen," Alex asked, in a slightly threatening tone before leaving, "don't get in the way with any personal plans I have for Brooke."

Watching him leave, Ellen confirmed in her mind that she did make a deal with the devil and now may have sacrificed Brooke MacIntosh to make the deal.

CHAPTER 36

❧

Kenny Thorton had some payments to make, along with recruiting some new agents to solicit for TTWC. He knew that these two tasks went hand to hand together as having his current staff of sales associates getting well paid in front of some potential recruits made his job easier, albeit more dangerous, as he carried large amounts of cash to these meetings. But he felt safe as he had his Glock shoved in his waistband and in plain view of his audience, who did not fear violence but respected those willing to use it.

The fact that Kenny would show up in an expensive car with a bag of cash reinforced to his associates and recruits that he was a white dude not to be fucked with. His first meeting was on the city's north side in an appropriately chosen place among the tombstones in Bellefontaine Cemetery, one of the oldest cemeteries in St. Louis.

The cemetery was also a national abortorium, one of a handful of cemeteries in the nation to earn that distinction. Here lay many of the families that started St. Louis and whose visions and financial fortunes made St. Louis one of the nation's great cities in the 1800s and early 1900s. Buried here were the great beer barons, including the Busch family, industrialists, architects, and inventors who were influential in the growth of St. Louis and the country. There were also influential politicians and authors whose rulings and writings shaped the nation's opinion of slavery and explorers, including William Clark, who, with Merriweather Lewis, explored and mapped the vast Louisiana Purchase territories. However, for his meeting place this morning, Kenny chose the site of one of the most recent cemetery residents, radio personality, and far-right shit disturber, Rush Limbaugh. Kenny found it ironic that Rush, who railed against the decay of urban America, placing the decline exclusively at the footsteps of democrats running the cities, would choose to be buried in this cemetery. While an oasis, it was in the middle of one of the most crime-ridden areas in St. Louis. So, as morbid as it seemed to walk through a cemetery, Kenny Thorton enjoyed the time he visited here. Also, ironically, not lost on Kenny was that he and Rush both shared an addiction to opioids. It was not what killed Rush Limbaugh directly, but the fact that both Rush and Kenny were addicts seemed to create a brotherhood between them.

Kenny also picked the Limbaugh family plot to provide a bit of history and context to Antonee and his bros, the men he would meet soon. Kenny always met Antonee at a different spot in the cemetery, making small talk about whose grave they were near. For his part, Antonee could give a shit about any old white crackers buried here. He was not interested in history as he was here to pick up his money and get the hell out because while Antonee was comfortable with death, especially the death of those administered by his hand, he was not comfortable in the cemetery. However, he knew the meeting place was a smart idea, being the safest area in a 2-mile radius. He knew Kenny would not meet at Antonee's crib, nor would meeting out in the open on the street be a better choice. Antonee knew those dangers and if anyone saw him meeting Kenny with his shiny white Audi parked nearby. They would assume Kenny was a cop, or word would get around that Kenny was moving some cash in Antonee's direction, and neither of them would survive the onslaught of bullets from a rival looking to make a score and a point. The cemetery was indeed the safest place for a meeting between a former opioid-addicted doctor turned insurance entrepreneur and a gang leader turned local businessman.

Kenny waited, looking at the headstones, the trees, and flowers, peacefully taking in the contrast of scenery between life and death. While

Kenny was not a long-range planner, he was seriously thinking of being buried here himself. This cemetery was one of the few places in St. Louis where you could choose to have a green, natural burial. Kenny liked the thought of naturally becoming compost. He always thought a bit more about his death after every meeting with Antonee or any of his recruits. Antonee was especially cold-hearted and ruthless. As if on cue, Kenny felt a chill as his skin tingled in heightened awareness as Antonee, along with two of his homies, all packing, suddenly appeared from behind a large mausoleum. Their stealth movements always shook Kenny, but he knew it was a skill for street survival that they faced every day.

They walked up to Kenny, who went to greet them with a handshake and chest hug.

"What's up, dawg?" Kenny said, dropping all pretense of proper English learned through his 24 years of very expensive, private, and medical school education.

Antonee pulled back with a look of disgust on his face as he hated when white people automatically reverted to hood lingo as if to make a connection. Antonee simply said, "All good, now let's get down to bidness as me, and my homies don't want to be here any longer than we be needing to."

"So, I take it no history lesson on who's grave we are standing by?" Kenny asked, knowing the answer was in the menacing stares by the three men, each tapping their pieces shoved in pants hanging halfway down their hips. "Do you want to introduce me to your friends?" Kenny added, knowing he was irritating Antonee, a man with a very short and dangerous fuse.

Flashing a sly smile, his surprisingly perfect white teeth glistening in the sun, Antonee said mockingly, "We will leave the introductions for our annual sales meeting in Hawaii. Ya, hear me, bruh?"

At that, all three laughed, or at least reduced their menacing glares, to help reduce the tension that always was part of these meetings.

"Ok, how many new contracts do you have for me this week, Antonee?" Kenny asked, getting down to business.

"We got us 12 new papers this week. That tells me you be owing $4800. You got that dawg?"

Handing over the policies to Kenny, Antonee added, "We got some more brothers interested in making some clean coin, so I be needing another $1000 to recruit them if that be all right with you, boss man?"

"Seems solid, Antonee. So, let's call it an even six large for the policies and the recruitment bonuses, then another 30% on the $4800, but to make it clean, I will give you $1500 for your cut."

Kenny knew that Antonee liked to always come out a little ahead, and besides, an extra couple of hundred was not going to break him or the company. These 12 policies would be worth millions of dollars to Alex Finnegan when they were cashed in. Kenny also knew the chances were 50/50 that Antonee would pay off any of his boys their actual cut. Kenny did not care who got paid or how much, as long as he got the policies. Stripping out $7,500 in hundred-dollar bills, he handed them to Antonee.

"You run into any questions about what you are doing selling these policies?" Kenny asked, aware of the importance of finding out if the word on the street was catching up to them.

"No, all good, bruh. Besides, everyone know better than to ask Antonee what he be working. Ain't none of their worry, and if they do start asking my boys here," pointing to his two guard dogs flanking him, he continued, "they get them straight out quick. You feel me?"

"All good, Antonee. Same time, same place, two weeks from now."

"We be here, K, and just so you know, bruh, I know what cracker be buried right here, below our feet, and I am glad he is. I don't give a shit about none of these other old dead white motherfuckers, but this cracker. I know the shit he say about us niggas, and I hope he enjoy all the homies pissing on his grave."

With that, both Antonee and Kenny walked away. Kenny headed off to his car parked near the entry of the cemetery and went to his next meet-up on the south side on Jefferson Avenue. Antonee and his bros went out a side gate and into the violent streets of north St. Louis. They may have physically lived in two different worlds, but they were intertwined in ways neither of them thought possible due to Alex Finnegan.

CHAPTER 37

After her dinner the previous evening with Angie Sullivan, Rhonda woke up the following morning with a killer hangover. Partly because of the large amount of booze she consumed and partly because all the information she was trying to process kept her from getting any sleep. She tossed and turned over what she knew, what she suspected, and most importantly, what she did not know. Her gut told her the carjackings and Audi were connected. She even suspected the carjackings were all done by the same people, but what she did not know was the biggest question of all. Why? She was thrown off by the fact that usually, carjackings were a random crime meets opportunity kind of thing and not well planned. The three murders the Audi was potentially part of seemed not random, almost planned, but she did not know if they were all connected.

A drug dealer in north St. Louis was murdered during a large gathering of neighborhood users, a female lawyer leaving work late at night, and a grandfather walking to his car from a Cardinals' game. Murders, if connected, were usually connected as a pattern of a gang war, revenge killing, or lover's quarrel. She also had the unsolved deaths of the junkie near Pappy's Restaurant, recently identified as Tayjon Reynolds, and the bicyclist Brian Coffman killed in Forest Park. She would push those aside for now since she saw no connection, primarily based on the cause of death, between those cases to the others. However, she would look more into the junkie's case as drug users, and their dealers sometimes overlap with murder. While it seemed hundreds, if not thousands, of the area's citizens were drug addicts, it always surprised her the overlapping connections between users and dealers. But she did not have time to chase down every link as she knew the streets would hand her several more murder cases to solve by the weekend. So, she would focus on what her gut told her: focus first on the white Audi. She also had Detective Sullivan and her team review all the area's carjackings to see if common trends or perpetrators popped up.

With her head still throbbing, Rhonda downed a second cup of black coffee, which had no effect at all on easing the pain. After rubbing her temple, she pulled up the white Audi's license plate, TTWC 21, in the DMV database.

Within seconds, as she had hoped, the Audi owner showed up as Kenneth Thorton on Westmoreland Street, St. Louis. While not knowing the house's exact location, Rhonda knew the neighborhood well. An area filled with stately homes behind locked gates on treelined and cobblestone streets. Like many in St. Louis, this neighborhood was a small pocket of protected old money, within earshot or, in some cases, gunshots, of areas that had seen better days. The location was no more than 15 minutes from Detective Simon's precinct. So, before leaving, she quickly texted Angie Sullivan, primarily to see how she was feeling this morning and to remind her to look at the other carjacking cases to see if she could make any other connections.

Detective Simon headed off west to the Central West End. This neighborhood made the national news as two gun-toting residents, a criminal defense lawyer Mark McCloskey and his wife Patricia, stood on their lawn with an AR–15 and a handgun pointing them towards a BLM protest movement passed by their home. The left, right, and the media all used the incident to raise the temperature a few more unnecessary degrees, which increased the animosity between citizens locally and nationally.

When does all the hatred between people end? Rhonda thought as she drove to Ken Thorton's house. Maybe society was doomed, and we were near the biblical end of days. It certainly seemed people had no regard for human life anymore, at least the people with whom she interacted. She pulled up to the house, and after parking on the street, she took a minute to survey the surroundings. Thorton's was a little on the small side as houses go in this neighborhood. However, with an imposing granite façade and its three stories, the house was anything but small to Rhonda. However, it was very rundown compared to the other homes on the street. Rhonda was sure the neighbors, and the neighborhood trustees, probably the same ones battling the McCloskey's over street rights, were none too happy with Mr. Kenneth Thorton. The sidewalk and driveway showed significant cracking. The landscape was sparse, with no color to speak off. What bushes the house had in front of it were overgrown and untrimmed. As she walked up the five granite stairs to the front porch, she noticed small things like the 10-foot-high windows having cracks in the panes and calking peeling from the frames. The paint was also peeling from the front door, where a newspaper collection had stacked up. If this house were not in one of the most prominent areas of St. Louis, she would think it was a crack house in a downtrodden neighborhood where so many homicides and drug deals occurred. However, she would not be surprised if this home was a crack house or drug haven, as she knew in her business the selling and using of drugs did not stop at specific zip codes.

Ringing the doorbell, she could hear the chimes echoing through the cavernous hallways as she glanced through the windows paralleling each side of the front door. There was no sound from inside after the first few seconds. She waited while slowly unbuckling her holster and laying her hand on her gun, as she did not know what she may be walking into or Kenny Thorton's state of mind. She rang the bell again, but this time she faintly heard footsteps. While still peering in the window, as soon as she saw who she assumed to be Kenny Thorton walking down the hallway, she backed away from the window so as not to give him cause for alarm or anger at the intrusion. She did not have a warrant and was only here to ask a few questions. She wanted to tread lightly to get Mr. Thorton talking as freely as possible.

Opening the door, coffee cup in hand, wearing a wrinkled Cardinals t-shirt and faded running shorts, was Kenneth Thorton. He looked as if he had just gotten up, and while it was morning, in Detective Simon's opinion, it was late enough in the morning for any decent person to have showered, shaved, and brushed their teeth. Kenny did not appear to have done any of these morning rituals.

"Yeah, what can I do for you?" Kenny gruffly asked as he rubbed his eyes, then his hands through his brown hair, which was so matted that it looked like it had not seen a shower and squirt of shampoo for a while.

"Mr. Thorton, Kenneth Thorton. I am Detective Rhonda Simon, St. Louis police department," she said as she showed him her badge.

Showing no interest in looking at the badge in any detail, but at the same time showing no sense of fear, anger, or concern most people do when talking to a cop, he simply said, "Nice to meet you, Detective. What can I do for you?"

"If you don't mind, I would like to ask you a few questions."

"Well, that depends on the questions, Detective. What is the subject matter, if I may ask?"

"Primarily your car, a 2019 white Audi A6, license plate TTWC 21," Rhonda replied.

With an understandably sudden rise in his voice, he immediately asked, "My car, what? Has it been stolen?" He hopped off the porch and walked to the driveway and garage on the right side of the house, where, to his relief, the car was still there.

Partially because her head still hurt and knowing the car was in the driveway as she saw when she drove up to the house, Detective Simon waited on the porch until Kenny returned.

"Ok, Mr. Thorton. Your car is obviously in your driveway, as you just ascertained. So, to answer your first question, no, it was not stolen. What I want to know is the whereabouts of your car on a couple of occasions recently and whether you were driving it at the time."

"Hmm," was all Kenny said. Detective Simon knew that this is when most people begin to clam up or act nervous, but Kenny merely said,

"Detective, I would love to answer your questions, but I need another cup of coffee. Can I get you one as well?"

Nodding yes, Kenny said, "If you would just wait out here on the porch, we could chat for a few minutes." He disappeared back into the house once she told him how she takes her coffee. She did not follow him as she knew it was unlawful for her to enter the house unless asked or she had a warrant. He did not seem to be a flight risk, so she sat on one of two Raton chairs on the porch. Besides, something about Kenny Thorton made her think she was dealing with someone who, while a bit frayed, was not uneducated. He had intelligence, but she also sensed he had experience dealing with cops.

After several minutes, while Rhonda looked around at the better-maintained homes occupied by Kenny's neighbors, he came out with two cups of coffee and several pastries on a tray.

"I thought you might be hungry, as well. My guess, Detective, is you wake up, down a cup of coffee or two, and normally skip breakfast? Am I right?"

He was right, and Rhonda was now sure Kenny Thorton had experience dealing with cops. Grabbing the coffee and a pastry, Rhonda thought it best just to ask away.

"So, Mr. Thorton."

"Please, Detective, call me Kenny."

"Ok, Kenny. Can you tell me, were you driving your car on the night of June 29th, approximately 8:30 p.m. near Olive and 8th street?"

"Umm, let me think," Kenny said, with no indication he was biding time to make up a story but instead trying to remember the date. Looking at his phone and scrolling what would seem to be his calendar, he replied, "That was a Tuesday night, and I was probably near the area coming back home from a Cardinals game."

Rhonda asked, "Pretty early to be coming back from a Cards game, isn't it? That would be about the 5th or 6th inning for a 7:00 start time."

Kenny answered, "Well, I can tell you are a fan, so you know what I mean when I say this. Wouldn't you leave early as lousy as they have been playing lately?"

Nodding, Detective Simon said, "You got me there, Kenny. I have left a few games early this year, too." Not wanting to get off subject, Rhonda then asked, "How about June 26th, around 9:00 p.m. near the vicinity south of the Stadium?"

"Well, Detective, you are finding out very quickly that I don't have much of a social life, but I am a huge baseball fan. On the 26th, I think it was Saturday night, I was going to a Cards game, and I like to park south of the stadium on surface lots because the traffic getting out is easier after the game."

Rhonda nodded, thinking for a minute. So far, she was getting nowhere.

"Detective, unless it is a crime going to Cardinals' games, I am not sure what you are after here?" Kenny asked.

Trying a different tactic, she pulled out a photo of a still video image of the three suspects involved in the carjacking and murder at the law offices. Showing him the picture, she asked, "I know this is not the best photo, but do you recognize any of these individuals?"

Taking the photo with no signal of surprise or concern, he studied it for a few seconds and handed it back to her. "No, Detective, I don't recognize those guys, and by the looks of them, I probably don't want to meet them in a dark alley."

"No, you don't," Rhonda replied.

"Again, Detective, I have to ask, what does any of this have to do with me or my car?"

Before answering that question, Rhonda asked, "Do you ever lend your car to anyone? Have you ever left the keys in it while you parked it at the stadium, or if you wanted to get out early, left the keys with a parking lot attendant you trusted and knew well?"

Pausing a second before answering, Kenny said, "Yeah, I know it is a stupid thing to do, but sure, sometimes when I know I am leaving early, and I don't want to be blocked, I flip the keys and an extra $20 to the guy to make sure he can move the car before anyone blocks me. You know, Detective, I just have a basic trust in people, and the worst that can happen is they go for a joy ride or bang up the car. It's just a replaceable machine, so no big deal."

"Or they could take the car and be involved in murder," Rhonda answered tersely.

The word murder got Kenny's attention. Sitting up, he asked, "What murder are you talking about, Detective?"

"Well, Kenny, we have two murders, both potentially involving car-jacking's on the 26th and 29th, the days you were at the Cardinals' game. On the 29th, we got your car with your plates in the area where a murder and carjacking occurred. On the 26th, we saw a car like your make, model, and color near the scene, but we did not get a clear view of the plates."

Kenny said nothing at first but took a deep breath. "You know, I read about both those murders. Tragic. It makes me sick, but I assure you, Detective, me and my car had nothing to do with those murders."

Rhonda was beginning to come to the same conclusion. She had lots of circumstantial evidence with many missing or un-connected pieces. But, Kenny was forthright about his car's whereabouts around the Cardinals games, not usually the approach a guilty person takes. While video footage existed of his vehicle near the scene on the 29th, there was no footage showing any contact with the suspects. On the 26th, there was video and visual footage of a white Audi interacting with two men before and after the Thomson murder. However, Rhonda had no footage of them committing the murder. And until Detective Sullivan or Rhonda compared videos from both murder scenes, she was not even sure the guys running away from her that night were the same guys in the law firm's parking lot after the Kim DeAngelo killing.

She asked one more question to evoke a reaction from him. "Kenny, do you know a man named William Burroughs?"

"Nope, never heard of him. Why?"

"Well, Mr. Burroughs, a known drug dealer, was shot to death about a month ago up in north St. Louis, and the only lead we have is a white Audi who dropped off two men at the house. Twenty minutes later, William Burroughs was killed."

Kenny got up from his chair and paced a bit before turning to Rhonda.

"Detective, I will assume you are very good at your job. I will further assume you asked me that question because before you came over for this visit, you googled me. If you did, you probably discovered I was a former doctor who lost my license due to opioid addiction and selling opioids on the street." His voice was rising still, "Now, you probably also know once an addict, always an addict, so when my license was revoked, you assumed I needed to get my fix on the street. And Detective, you are right on that, but that was years ago, and now, thank God, I am clean. So, don't try to connect these bullshit dots around me. I have lost my wife, my money, and my profession. I know I will be labeled an addict for life, but now I am not addicted to anything."

Rhonda was impressed by his speech but did not believe a word of it. She thought he was still using based on how he looked this morning and the mention of William Burroughs certainly got Kenny a little more animated than he was previously.

"Mr. Thorton, no dots will be connected that don't have a reason to, but I am trying to solve a few murders before the next one lands on my desk, and I have to turn over every rock. Then I will be on my way. I have one more question. You drive a nice enough car, and this house, while rundown, probably has utility bills higher than most people's monthly mortgages. So, my question is: what do you do for money? How do you make a living?"

"Detective, while I think you are getting way over your skis, I will answer that question because I deeply respect cops and the job you do. Living here, we know you guys are the big blue wall that keeps us safe. I own an insurance company called TTWC. You know that because you know my license plate, which is the company's name."

"What does it stand for?" Rhonda asked.

"Their Time Will Come," Kenny replied.

"Kind of a morbid name, Kenny."

"Not morbid, Detective. Feta Compli. All life ends. Sometimes peacefully, sometimes accidentally, and sometimes violently, as you know all too well in your job. And when it does, you or your loved ones will be glad you had some insurance."

Handing him her empty cup of coffee, Rhonda handed him her card and walked down the porch stairs. "Kenny, piece of advice. Don't give your keys to any parking lot attendants. Not a smart move."

Rhonda got in her car and drove a few hundred yards before doing a U-turn in the street as she wanted to take in the neighborhood once again. As she passed Kenny's house again, he stood, seemingly unfazed, on the porch, and he gave her a nod and a wave as she passed by. Once out of site, Kenny punched in the numbers to Alex's untraceable burner phone and entered a code that he knew would signal Alex. He needed to meet with him the following afternoon. A return code came back from Alex, indicating Alex had accepted the meeting.

As Rhonda drove away, she thought there were way too many red flags to eliminate Kenny as having a significant involvement in these murders. She was also troubled by how quickly he recalled the murders when Rhonda had not mentioned Kim DeAngelo or Bill Thomson's names. Kenny had to refer to his calendar and think about his whereabouts, but the mention of unnamed murders triggered his recall instantly.

CHAPTER 38

B rooke had just finished her morning shift and headed to the hospital cafeteria to get lunch. After making her food choice and grabbing an iced tea at the drink dispenser, she headed to a small table but stopped hearing a familiar voice. She looked over to see one of her former high school classmates, Allison Quillen, who had gone on to medical school, waving her over to her table.

Putting her tray on the table, Brooke and Allison embraced as it had been over two years since they had last seen each other.

"Allison, what are you doing here?" was Brooke's first question. "I thought you were doing your residency in Nashville?"

"I was, but I am back. Nashville was great, but I missed the fam, so I moved back."

"And you are working here?" Brooke said while lifting and looking at Allison's badge to confirm her question.

"Yep. Working in the emergency room. You know me, Brooke, love to be where the action is."

Brooke knew that about Allison. They had grown up in the same neighborhood, had both gone to Visitation Academy, and while they were not in the same circle of close friends, their paths crossed enough at parties and social events around town. While Brooke was a more intro-spective thinker and planner, Allison loved to jump right into anything that sounded fun, challenging, or risky. The ER suited Allison perfectly as she loved the intensity of life or death happening around her hour by hour. Especially in an ER as busy as the one in Barnes. Being in the center of the city and a Level 1 trauma center, her ER got most of the violent crime and horrific accident cases in the St. Louis area.

"I understand you are doing great up on the transplant floor. That is perfect for you, Brooke. You always loved the interaction with patients and their families, but I bet you still get too close to them, don't you? Still taking your work home with you every day, am I right?" Allison asked.

Brooke smiled warmly at Allison, knowing she pegged Brooke correctly. Brooke said, "You know me too well, Allison. I love what I do. I love getting to know the patients and their families and the joy they feel when they get a transplant."

"Yeah, I don't see much joy down in the ER. I see so much violence, anguish, tears, and death. I see the stupidity and savagery of humans. It sometimes makes me sick, but it is so short-term that I don't have time to think of my patients as they are in, out, or gone within hours. So, I don't get emotionally attached, which is not my strong suit, as you know."

Brooke nodded in agreement. She knew she and Allison were in the right places for their personalities. They spent the rest of lunch catching up on families, shared friends, and lovers lost or still being pursued.

Allison then said, "I have to ask you, has anything changed with the transplantation protocols and processes lately?"

"No, still too many people need organs, and not enough get them. That seems like such an odd question. Why do you ask?"

"Well, as you know, we get our share of crazies in the ER. Whether crazy because of illegal drugs these folks are on, legal drugs they are off but need to back on, or just crazy with grief, we have recently had some whacked out family members."

"Sounds like a normal day or night in your world," Brooke responded.

"Yeah, for the most part, normal, but over the last several weeks, we have had a couple of incidences that would seem to connect my crazies with your transplant floor."

"How so?" Brooke asked.

"Well, twice, we had two unrelated patients, both gunshot victims, die, and the mother, or grandmother, hard to say, kept yelling about getting their money. I did not think much about it since I had my hands full, but I assumed they were talking about getting the possessions back from the deceased."

"That makes sense. Many of these folks don't trust banks, and they carry lots of cash on them. Maybe that is why they were both murdered, I guess. They probably also don't trust the hospital handling those possessions," Brooke's added.

"I thought the same thing," Allison said, "but when things calmed down a bit, I overheard both women yelling to whoever would listen that they "paid the policy, and they wanted their $50,000.""

"Insurance money?" asked Brooke. "What an odd time to think about that, but I guess shock had them all messed up. And they both said the same amount, $50,000, right?"

"Yep, the same amount of money. And here is the other weird thing, and why I asked about anything going on upstairs on your floor. Both women talked about they needed to get their boys to The Center to get their parts out. They kept saying The Center, so they could get paid."

Brooke said nothing, but she could feel her face freeze up, her eyes in a distant glaze.

"Brooke, Brooke, what is going on? You have a weird look in your eyes. Does any of this make sense to you?"

Snapping out of her transfixed state, Brooke composed herself. With a forced laugh, she looked at Allison and said, "Who knows? As you said, it is cray-cray down there, and I have no idea what those women were talking about."

Sensing the mood had lightened a bit, Allison laughed lightly as well. "You're right, Brooke. Cray-cray doesn't even describe what goes on down in the ER. But you know, the crazier the shit gets, the more I love it."

As they both got up with their trays to take them to the trash area, they agreed to get together for drinks and dinner very soon. After a quick goodbye hug, Brooke turned to Allison and said, "Hey, if you get any other crazed family members talking like this again, send me a text. I might want to come down and see what is up with them. I may not like the crazy as much as you do, Allison, but I could use a good mystery to solve."

Allison agreed, and they both went to their separate elevator banks to get back to work. Brooke, for her part, thumbed through her phone and looked at phone numbers for both Alex Finnegan and Ellen Calabrese. Before dialing either, she wondered who would be the most honest in answering her questions. By the time the elevator door opened, she had her answer. She texted Dr. Calabrese for a meeting because she knew that while Dr. Calabrese was a direct, hard charger, no-nonsense doctor, she was not full of bullshit like she felt Alex Finnegan was and who seemed to relish it.

CHAPTER 39

Around 11:00 a.m. and a few hours before Alex met with Kenny Thornton, he texted Ellen asking her to swing by his office before noon.

Knocking politely on the door frame to announce her arrival at his office, Ellen walked in right as Alex was just finishing a call, giving Ellen a circling of his index finger, indicating that he would be wrapping up in just a minute. While Alex was on the call, Ellen walked over to his wall of fame, as he called it, to read over the many articles, citations, and plaques Alex had gotten over the years. She had scanned all of this before but was always impressed with all Alex had accomplished. However, she knew through her dealings with him, and successful men like him, most eventually screw up because the success they achieved, the power they had, made them invincible and above it all in their minds. That is why most men, based on the history of the gender, took high risks in business and relationships because they felt they would never fail. And, of course, many hid their digressions throughout their lives. Still, many more ended up divorced multiple times, disgraced in the business community, or the worst of decisions and outcomes, eventually landing in prison for various white-collar crimes. Alex was not married, so he could not screw that up, though Ellen knew he viewed women as disposable. She wondered what Alex's downfall would be. She knew he would have one. His ego was too large to avoid it. She just needed to make sure he did not drag her down with him. Hearing him end his conversation, she turned back from the wall and sat down.

"What's up, Alex?"

"What's up is I have banks, lawyers, investors, regulators up my ass 24/7. That's what's up."

"Well, at least you don't have a woman breaking your balls or crushing your heart, right?"

Alex laughed, "Well, you do a pretty good job breaking my balls. Thank God you can't break my heart, as well."

"Alex, we all know you don't have a heart, but I appreciate the compliment on me being a ball breaker. I kind of like that role. Now, what can I do for you?"

"Well, I just wanted to let you know that I investigated Frank Esposito's situation, and unfortunately, I can't think of any way we can help him. He will have to trust the system will find him a match soon because he is a very sick man."

Quietly, Ellen said, "Thank you for looking into it. I was not optimistic that we could do anything, but it was worth a try."

Sounding very sincere, Alex consoled Ellen by saying, "Sorry, but if it was a year from now and we were operating as I think we will be, we could probably save him, using the resources we are bringing to this problem." Then adding with a dramatic emphasis, "Damn, Ellen. This is why it is so damn important that we are successful and change the paradigms of transplants. We can't help your brother-in-law, but together you and I, hopefully, will shake this industry up and save a lot of people who need transplants."

Ellen left Alex's office thinking that maybe she saw a bit of humanity in Alex for the first time. For his part, Alex, while watching Ellen go, he thought he had just put on a fabulous acting job. It got the desired effect of Ellen's empathy and increased loyalty to him.

What Ellen did not know and would hopefully never know is that Alex planned to use Frank Esposito's situation as a case history of what The Center could do and how it will save many more lives. Using the complete resources and technology from the GUTS command center,

Alex identified all potential future donors who were perfect matches for Frank Esposito. Unfortunately, all of them were still alive, but if any of them died in time to save Frank Esposito, Alex would prove his concept that people would do anything for love or money. He just needed an unsuspecting ally or dupe to prove this.

As Alex prepared for his next meeting, he knew his plan needed to be executed quickly as Frank Esposito probably had only weeks to live. While he could care less if Frank got new lungs, Alex saw this as a perfect opportunity to test the loyalties of those once again on his payroll. Plus, he hoped to make Vinnie Calabrese look like a fool, or worse.

CHAPTER 40

Alex and Kenny met at their usual location, the base of King Louis IX's statue in Forest Park. Kenny's message seemed somewhat urgent, especially since they had just met recently to update Kenny's progress with TTWC. So, Alex, curious about the news and pressed for time, waded right in.

"Kenny, what was so urgent you needed to see me?"

"What was so urgent was that I had a visit from a cop yesterday, Detective Rhonda Simon, who was asking about random carjackings and murders that had happened recently," Kenny said.

"Ok," said Alex. "Unless you have moved up from opioid addiction to carjacking and murder, why was she seeing you?"

"She claimed my car was spotted and confirmed to be nearby at least one of the three crimes, as well as possibly being near the other two crimes," Kenny answered.

"Well, was it nearby? Were you involved in any of this, Kenny?"

"Me? Personally? No. I wasn't, but I am not sure my car wasn't near each crime scene."

Eyeing Kenny now very suspiciously, as he knew all drug addicts, including Kenny, were habitual liars, Alex probed harder and said, "Kenny, what the fuck does that mean? Why would your car be near these crime scenes, but you weren't?"

Looking down and casually kicking the dirt beneath his shoes, Kenny responded, "Um, well, sometimes I let some of my crew use the car. It helps them be seen in a nice car to attract more recruits and legitimize the business."

"Your crew?" Alex asked incredulously. "Your crew are a bunch of thugs and criminals who would have no problems stealing your car and cutting your throat. Do you have them over for Saturday afternoon BBQs at your house as well?"

Kenny said nothing as he knew best just to let Alex vent and not try to defend his actions.

"Kenny, besides incredibly stupid judgment and the possibility of being an accessory to a crime, if your crew was involved, how was it left with the cop?"

"I told her, when I am at the Cards games, I sometimes leave my keys with parking lot attendants, and she believed that, I guess. She can't tie me to any of the crimes, and frankly, she cannot connect my car to the suspects committing the crimes. She just told me to quit letting people borrow my car."

"Yeah. I agree with that."

"One more thing, though," Kenny added. "She asked about TTWC."

"How the hell would she know about TTWC?"

"Um, it is my vanity plate on my car."

"Shit, Kenny. Why the hell would you have that as your vanity plate? We are trying to be low-key about this. Remember?"

"Well, I figured that having it registered on something official like my plates at the DMV would help us legitimize the business with my crew and help me recruit. Besides, I get kind of a kick out of being President of the company, and you know, maybe helping grow it into something I can be proud of. You know, Alex, it has been a long time since I had any meaning or focus in my life, and TTWC is something real to me. Besides, all the cop knows is we sell insurance. She did not ask anything more about it, but it's out there."

With anger building up in him, Alex got closer to Kenny, grabbing his shirt collar, and whispering so no one could hear them, "Kenny, I don't give a fuck about you gaining meaning in your life. I don't give a shit about TTWC as a business. I don't care about TTWC's customers or your crew. TTWC exists only for The Center and me. Kenny, lucky for you, I have all our tracks covered and have set up the company perfectly and legitimately, so even if it's out there, it will pass any scrutiny if the cops start sniffing around."

Kenny firmly took Alex's hands off his collar and stared him down as two prize fighters glared during a weigh-in ceremony. Kenny said, "Alex, I appreciate everything you have done for me, but don't forget the sacrifice I made to keep your career going, taking the heat for you, and losing everything because of that. So don't ever fucking touch me again, you prick."

Physically Alex knew that Kenny, with rage boiling up inside, could take down Alex easily, so Alex tried to diffuse the situation before it got out of hand.

"Kenny, you are right, and maybe when this is over, and The Center does not need TTWC anymore, we will spin it off, and it will be a legit, standalone business that will be all yours. No involvement with me whatsoever. Your baby to grow and do whatever you want to. How does that sound?"

"Sounds like you are afraid I will kick your ass here and now. It sounds like you are afraid I can have my crew cap your ass whenever I want. It sounds like my old friend Alex is backed in a corner and promising anything to save his ass. That is what it sounds like to me."

"Ok, let's just get back on the plan here. What happened with the cop, your car, is all behind us, and I don't see that being a problem, but I have another assignment for you."

After explaining the assignment, Alex gave Kenny an envelope with $10,000 and said, "Just a little something to help on the project. Use it as you see fit."

Holding onto the envelope, as Alex walked away, Kenny was glad he did not mention that he thought he recognized the suspects shown to him by Detective Simon in the Kim DeAngelo murder. Currently, Antonee and his crew were murderers and some of the top producers for

TTWC. He also did not tell Simon that all three of the murder victims had a connection to both he and Alex. Kenny knew he was in trouble, but he would sit on this information for a while until he could determine how to use the information to best save his ass or maybe bury Alex's if needed.

CHAPTER 41

Rhonda Simon's phone rang, and looking down at it, she saw it was a call from Angie Sullivan.

"Hey, Sully. What's up?"

"Living the dream, Rhonda, living the dream. Before I get too whimsical about this damn great life we lead, I wanted to give you an update on our search of carjacking crimes that may have had a similar M.O. as your cases, along with any sightings of a mysterious white Audi."

"And? Anything?"

"Well, no to the perps and the white Audi. We have had plenty of carjackings in the area in the last six months, but for the most part, different perps in most jacks, random locations in the city and the county, and with random victims. Also, despite nearly 30 jacks, there was only one other murder. You remember the one where the young mother was grocery shopping, and they jacked and offed her with her baby still in the car?"

"Yeah, I remember that one," Rhonda said. "Sent chills down my spine that a young woman doing something as normal as grocery shopping gets killed for a joy ride. Thank God they abandoncd the car when they found the baby there."

Angie responded, "We got those assholes. I hope they get the jumbo-sized lethal injection down in Potosi."

Knowing she still had a ton of work to do, Rhonda tried to wrap up the call thanking Angie for her help, but Angie stopped her.

"Hold on, Rhonda. Before you think all my efforts are for naught, you may have forgotten for a minute that my three favorite things are yapping, drinking, and trying to get laid, and sometimes not all in that order," Sully said, laughing.

"Well, you do have your priorities correctly in order, Sully. So, how do your debauchery lifestyle and my unsolvable cases connect?"

"The other day, after reviewing all the carjacking cases, I went down to Malone's, and as the booze got flowing, so did my mouth. I was working on a potential candidate for my bed that evening and casually mentioned to him what you and I were working on. Surprisingly, not only was my prince charming, ruggedly handsome, he had a memory like an elephant."

"How so? What did the future fourth Mr. Angie Sullivan have to say?" Rhonda asked.

"Not looking for another husband, my dear Rhonda. I just use them by the hour now. It makes it much easier. Anyway, what he said, and damn if I can remember his name now, was that he recalled both the DeAngelo lawyer murder and the old man murder near the ballpark."

"So, he reads the paper. So what?" responded Rhonda.

"I am not even sure he can read, and I certainly don't care if he does, but he did remember that both the lawyer and what was his name, Thomson, the old guy that got killed near Busch Stadium, worked on some high-profile drug cased a few years back. DeAngelo was a prosecuting attorney, and Thomson ran a pretty successful private investigation firm." Sully said with proudness in her voice that she remembered all the details.

On the other end of the phone, Rhonda was silent. Angie Sullivan let her percolate as she knew the wheels were turning in her head when Rhonda was quiet.

Finally, Rhonda said, "Sully, I am so glad you are a slutty drunk and met this guy. I never thought of connecting the victims. They seemed so random, so unconnected."

"Thank you, Rhonda. I take that as a compliment," laughed Angie, as did Rhonda. "Anything else I can do for you on these, just let me know. I have a gut feeling that if the victims are connected, so are the perps."

With promises of getting together soon, Rhonda ended the call, grabbed a piece of paper, and wrote the word 'DRUGS' on it. As widespread as drugs were in society, Rhonda knew there always seemed to be remote connections. She also wrote two names: Kim DeAngelo and William Thomson, then drew a line connecting them and added "shared cases." After thinking for a few more minutes, she wrote the name William Burroughs, dealer, and added a dotted line connecting him to DeAngelo and Thomson with a big question mark. As she thought about it more, she added one more name: Tayjon Reynolds. The overdose victim found dead in his car. She did not connect his name to the other three but put question marks next to his name. She then stared at the paper, wondering how or if, these four people were connected. She silently cursed what Angie had found. While it might get Rhonda closer to solving the crime, it also meant she was at a new starting point, which meant more long hours to her already long 10-hour days.

CHAPTER 42

V innie looked down at his phone and saw a text from a number he did not recognize. The message was a mystery, as it said: "Meet at Boat House, 8:00 a.m. re: Frank Esposito. No names." Vinnie had no idea what the text meant or who he was meeting, but obviously, someone knew that he was related to Frank and knew Frank's condition would ensure Vinnie would show up. At 8:00 a.m., the Boat House, a popular destination fronting the 22-acre Grand Lagoon in Forest Park, was usually empty as the restaurant's breakfast crowd was small. Most of the activity came later in the day when visitors, usually couples, would rent out the paddle boats and meander through the lagoon under small bridges and pathways nestled below the shadow of the Art Museum. It was one of the most beautiful and tranquil parts of the park. Vinnie knew that while most paddle boaters started their trip with love and romance in their eyes, they came back tired and angry at each other as paddle boats were notoriously difficult to paddle. Usually, one person did the lion's share of the paddling. He and Ellen had tried out the boats once, only once, which he suspected was the frequency shared by most of the visitors.

Arriving a few minutes before 8:00, he quickly found the person he was meeting dressed in a vintage St. Louis Rams jersey with the name "Bruce" stenciled on the back. Vinnie walked up next to the man, and as instructed, he said, "I am here for Frank Esposito."

It had been nearly seven years since the Rams left St. Louis, and the way they left, with corporate greed getting its way, reduced the number of fans still sporting jerseys. Most Rams jerseys, if not used as rags to wash your car, were now probably given away to shelters to clothe the homeless, and Vinnie's contact that morning certainly looked homeless or maybe worse.

The man turned to him, took out a piece of paper, handed it to Vinnie, and said, "Here are four perfect donor matches for Frank Esposito. Use it as you wish, but if you tell anyone of its existence or ask questions about it, you will find yourself becoming an organ donor sooner than you may have thought." With that, the man took off in a slight jog but not a hurried run around the lagoon, and in 30 seconds, he disappeared.

Vinnie sat down on a nearby bench and looked at the list. It had four people's names, addresses, phone numbers, emails, and medical information. Vinnie thought in his gut that Ellen had something to do with getting him this list, but it seemed so unethical that he was unsure why Ellen would risk her professional status to help him. Maybe that is why she used an intermediary. Ellen did say she would talk to Finnegan about what help he could provide. Maybe Finnegan had his hand in this, but Finnegan and Vinnie never liked each other. So, Vinnie thought Finnegan was less likely to help him than Ellen. Regardless of the list's source, Vinnie was glad he had it but was troubled. What was he supposed to do now that he had, perhaps, the key to Frank's life in his hands? Was he supposed to contact each of these people and ask them how close they were to dying? He chuckled to himself about how that conversation would go. He said out loud, "Hello, you don't know me, but I was wondering how close you think you are to dying and donating your lungs?" Click.

Vinnie then thought of talking to Frank and Sue about the list but quickly ruled that out because as sick as Frank was, he would never take advantage of others so he could live. Plus, they lived by such a strong moral code, much stronger than Vinnie's, that they would insist Vinnie report the list to the proper medical or law enforcement authorities. Vinnie then thought about something that always haunted him in his life. While he had been relatively successful, he also felt part of his life was incomplete. He would tell whoever would listen that he had never done anything significant with his life, but before dying, he would. Most of his friends thought he was nuts, but this lack of greatness, or maybe significance, haunted Vinnie. His failed marriage to Ellen and his strained relationship with his adult children reinforced his belief that he was a failure. Soon Vinnie looked at his phone and realized he had been sitting on the bench for nearly an hour, but he was still unsure what his next steps with the list would be.

CHAPTER 43

Ellen and Brooke had agreed to meet the following day over coffee at the Starbucks in Maryland Plaza in the Central West End. Close enough to both the hospital and The Center but not so close that they would risk the chance of being seen by nosey colleagues. Brooke assumed Ellen would follow up on the conversation and job offer she and Alex had the other night over dinner. Brooke was undoubtedly interested in understanding more about it. As much as she loved her job, the money Alex had proposed would not only help Brooke financially but would allow Brooke to help her parents, whose restaurant was still struggling. Brooke also wanted to see if Ellen reacted to the mention of The Center by the two women Allison overheard in the E.R.

At 7:00 a.m., the Starbucks had its usual crowd, and when Brooke arrived, she saw Ellen waving her over to her table. Before she headed over, Brooke went to the counter and ordered a skinny latte, then sat down with Ellen, who was slowly dipping her tea bag into her cup as she waited for the tea to steep. Brooke always considered herself a stylish dresser, and being physically fit, she wore clothes very well. She always admired how well Ellen looked every time she met her.

Brooke would describe Ellen's wardrobe and demeanor as stylish, elegant, and classy but not stuffy. While Brooke's mother was her role model in life, Brooke could see Ellen being a role model or mentor for her career. It was one of the things that attracted Brooke to the job offer at The Center. Ellen could be the difference-maker in accepting the job, and the buffer between Brooke and Dr. Finnegan, whom Brooke assumed would eventually want to get into her pants, like every other powerful man she met.

After exchanging morning pleasantries, Ellen got down to business. Usually, getting down to business was Ellen's style, but it was probably more urgent at 7:00 a.m. on a workday. Brooke assumed Ellen had a very full schedule.

"Brooke, Alex told me about your conversation with him and his presentation of our job offer to be Director of Transplant Synergy. I know it has only been a few days, but what is your initial reaction to our offer and you joining us at The Center?"

"Well, to be honest with you, I was taken aback, not necessarily by getting an offer, because I sensed that all of the meetings seemed like a job interview, and for the most part, you confirmed that. However, the salary doubles what I currently make. It certainly seems like a lot of money."

"It is a lot of money, and the position is vitally important. Also, don't forget the stock options because while the salary will make your life more comfortable, the stock options, if exercised, could make you a very wealthy young woman."

Brooke inhaled and exhaled deeply, took this all in, and prepared herself for the next question she was about to ask Ellen.

"Dr. Calabrese, I appreciate this opportunity, and while I have a general understanding of the job described by Dr. Finnegan, I know I have to accept the job before I get all the details in my role."

"That's right. I have the offer paperwork here," Ellen said as she pulled out a four-page document from her portfolio. She slid the paper to Brooke, who began to scan it over but did not ask for a pen to sign it.

"Dr. Calabrese, do you mind if I talk to my parents about the offer and have them look this over, including the NDA and non-compete components? I know these things are standard, but I always like to talk to my parents about big decisions like this. I promise I will get back to you next week."

"Brooke, that is fine. I wish my parents were still around as I always valued their opinion." Ellen finished her tea and began organizing her possessions, signaling the conversation was ending. Ellen started to stand up, and as she reminded Brooke to call her if she had any questions, the question Brooke asked soon had Ellen sitting down again.

"Dr. Calabrese, I do have one question, and it is going to sound odd." Ellen just smiled. It seemed every meeting with Brooke ended up with an odd question.

"Are you and Dr. Finnegan in any way aiding in the death of people to get more donors?"

"Wow, that is an odd question," Ellen replied, holding back her shock, then composing herself. "Are you asking because of our ideas on the choice of death decisions? Because if you are, we are not making those decisions. The patient is. That is what choice is all about."

Brooke sized up Ellen's demeanor and decided to wade into this subject slowly. After all, she had new information that neither Ellen nor Dr. Finnegan had brought up in past conversations, and if she was going to work with these people, she needed to know if they were truthful, or worse, criminals.

"I understand that you are letting the patient choose, and while perhaps this may be viewed as unethical and illegal in some circles, I understand that you are doing this to challenge the status quo. You are pushing to change our culture and laws. I respect that, and I think I might agree, but that is not what I am talking about."

Now with a look of puzzlement, but not complete surprise, assuming what Brooke's next question may be, Ellen asked, "So, what then are you talking about?"

"I have a friend who works in the E.R. at Barnes, and she told me the other day that two women, whose sons had died in a separate shooting and a stabbing, were both yelling and screaming about getting their money. They mentioned $50,000 from The Center or a center. My friend was unsure, and, of course, it was a hectic scene, as you might expect. Dr. Calabrese, do you think the women were talking about the Arch City Transplant Center?"

Looking at the employment contract sitting between them and knowing she should only reveal certain aspects of the business to employees under an NDA, Ellen took the safe route for now.

"I have no idea what those women were talking about. I assure you it has nothing to do with our Center. You know how shock affects people when faced with tragedy. They say crazy, unintelligible things. Center could mean anything, or it could mean nothing at all. A community center, a church, a bank, a person's name. Who knows?"

Eyeing Ellen more warily and thinking she was hiding something, Brooke decided to let the matter drop until she had more information. She responded to Ellen by saying, "That is what I told my friend." Brooke purposely kept Allison's name out of the conversation. "We both called it crazy talk."

Wanting to end the conversation, Ellen then got up quickly and told Brooke she had to run, busy day and all, and off she went, but before she did, Ellen pointed to the employment contract and said, "Please look that over as soon as you can. We want you on board so we can share our entire vision with you."

Brooke believed Ellen had a busy day, but she sensed her questions spooked Ellen. Hell, they frightened Brooke, too. *Just what were Doctors Calabrese and Finnegan up to?* Brooke thought to herself as she watched Ellen walk away.

CHAPTER 44

Detective Simon got to work trying to connect the multiple carjacking cases, not on the potential perps, or presence of the Audi, but any links to the victims. Most of what she needed to research would be found easily, but depending on how far back she would have to go, it could take some time. First, she would investigate the personal life and career of Kim DeAngelo, the lawyer murdered in the garage of her law firm's offices. She always hated researching those who were murdered because she often read about innocent people minding their own business at the time of the murder. In many cases, they were contributors to society, leaving great families and kids behind, all for something trivial, like a stolen car.

Kim DeAngelo's background was as Rhonda suspected it would be. Local girl, raised in affluent West St. Louis Country. After high school, she went on to DePauw University, then taking a slight career detour, she chose to go into a Teach for America program, where the best and brightest college graduates committed to two years of teaching in underserved communities. Ms. DeAngelo decided on the mean streets of North Philadelphia to teach.

After her Teach for America gig was over, she stayed in Philly, going to law school at Temple. Finally, putting her educational pursuits behind her, she graduated at 26 years of age, doing more at that young age than most people do in 50 years. After law school, she moved back to St. Louis to work as a prosecuting attorney for the city of St. Louis, where she stayed for five years. Then to make some serious money, she went on to the private sector, working at McConnell and McGrath, the firm she was at when she was murdered. Rhonda knew she would have to begin combing the archives of cases DeAngelo worked on as a prosecuting attorney. Then also, whether willing or not, get answers from a partner at McConnell and McGrath to understand what cases DeAngelo might have worked on there. Based on her experience, Rhonda knew that if there was a connection to a murder, it likely happened on a case DeAngelo worked on while a prosecuting attorney versus a case at the private law firm.

Then she looked up Bill Thomson, shot outside of Busch Stadium. Mr. Thomson, like Ms. DeAngelo, also had an impressive background. After graduating college at Mizzou, Mr. Thomson joined the Army, where he prospered, Rhonda guessed, for nearly 20 years as he rose to the rank of Captain. The units where Thomson worked were described in general terms, but Rhonda had enough experience in military operations and lingo that she rightfully assumed Mr. Thomson worked in special services. After leaving the military, Thomson went to D.C., where he spent ten years in cyber intelligence either for the CIA, NSA, or FBI, as the bio was vague about which agency Thomson worked. Mr. Thomson probably went from shooting the bad guys at point-blank range to finding their whereabouts through cyber snooping and ordering others to kill. At age 52, after government work, he joined the private sector by starting a firm called SCOPE. The firm was not a one-person detective operation taking photos of cheating husbands but a very sophisticated business described on its website as "using digital footprints to find the perpetrators of crime and corruption in the C-suite." Mr. Thomson's firm specialized in white-collar crime. At 65, Mr. Thomson sold his firm to unknown buyers, probably Rhonda assumed, for millions of dollars.

The first step was to find any connection between cases worked on by Kim DeAngelo as a special prosecutor, or at her law firm, to any cases worked on by SCOPE. She had a friend in the prosecutor's office, so that would not be any problem researching the department's cases while

DeAngelo worked there. To research clients SCOPE may have had in the overlapping time, she would have to find someone at SCOPE willing and able to talk—someone who would have worked with Thomson and was devasted by the news of his death. Using LinkedIn, she looked at all current SCOPE staff members whose LinkedIn network might have had connections to past employees of SCOPE, who by this time would be retired or moved on from the company, hopefully with no NDA in place. Sure enough, she found several former SCOPE employees, now retired and still living in St. Louis. She wrote down several possible names and their contact information. She would follow up with them over the next several days once she had gotten a list of cases DeAngelo worked on.

In the old days on the force, police work uncovered one physical clue at a time, such as a bullet casing or a blood sample. In many ways, that is still critical, but the modern cop knew that the real clues were often found in digital information or footprints. Rhonda felt that would be the key to solving these cases. She needed a baseline of cases or clients to share with the former SCOPE employee to see if they sounded familiar.

CHAPTER 45

After meeting with Ellen, Brooke went to work and noticed a text from Allison on her phone. It said: "Come down to the E.R. It must have been a full moon last night b/c cray-cray is back."

Brooke first ensured all her cases were in good shape and let her team know she would make a quick visit to the E.R. to help a friend out. They knew to text her if she was needed.

Brooke looked for Allison before heading into the main E.R. but then heard her in an exam room.

"Ma'am, please calm down. You are not helping matters with your son," Allison pleaded with the woman as she tried to steer her out of the exam room where her son lay dying of a gunshot wound.

Brooke entered the room as Allison and the woman got more involved in a battle of wills and strength, each pushing the other in and out of the exam room.

"Allison, what is her name?" Brooke quickly asked as she tried to intervene.

"I think Reynolds. That is what a friend of her kid told us before he ran off. He said he would call Mama Reynolds, and then she showed up 20 minutes later."

Grabbing the woman by the shoulder, softly but firmly, Brooke looked her in the eye and said calmly, "Mrs. Reynolds, please let the doctors and nurses work on your son. They are trying to help him."

"My boy, my boy!" Mrs. Reynolds cried out. "Ashari, hold on, son, hold on. Your mama is here. Your mama is here," she yelled as Brooke finally got control of her and guided her out of the exam room and into a side office near the main reception area.

Brooke sat her down while holding her hand and said, "Mrs. Reynolds, I am Brooke MacIntosh, and I work here at the hospital. I will stay with you while the doctors and nurses work on your son, work on Ashari."

Sobbing for a few minutes more, not talking, Mrs. Reynolds eventually looked at Brooke and said, "If you a doctor or a nurse, you should be in with my boy, not out with me. Be in with Ashari, be in there to help him."

"I am a nurse, Mrs. Reynolds, but I don't work in E.R., so I can't assist, and besides, the team in there is the best to help Ashari."

"So, why are you here with me? Are you a social worker? You with the police?"

"No, ma'am. As I said before, I am a nurse and work here at the hospital, but I work on the transplant floor. I was just here to visit my friend Allison, and I tried to help out."

Looking intently at Brooke with confusion in her eyes, Mrs. Reynolds whispered, "If you on the transplant floor, then you done know Ashari is going to die, and you want his parts when he gone."

"No, Mrs. Reynolds. That would never be something the hospital or I would do. Ashari is in good hands, and they will do everything they can for him."

"Well, if he do die, I signed all the paperwork. You get his parts, and I get the money, but I don't want the money. I want Ashari. He and his brother are all I got," Mrs. Reynolds yelled out.

Brooke thought for a minute and realized why Allison had texted her. Mrs. Reynolds might have said the same thing to Allison as the other mothers who saw their sons die several days ago.

"Mrs. Reynolds, listen to me. Just think about Ashari living a long, wonderful life with you and his brothers. Can you do that, Mrs. Reynolds?"

"I can do that, but his older brother, Tayjon, got murdered, and he died without me getting any money because he did not get taken to The Center fast enough to use his parts. I don't want Ashari to die, but I need the money if he does. That's why I signed the papers for him and his brothers. On the streets like they do, they more likely be dying than living."

Wondering if Mrs. Reynolds was talking coherently, Brooke decided she was stable enough to push for more answers, especially about the papers she signed and the money. Brooke used her position on the transplant floor to get Mrs. Reynolds to talk a bit more.

"Mrs. Reynolds, in case Ashari dies, and I pray he does not so that we handle him properly, can you show me the paperwork you signed? Do you have it on you?"

"Yeah, I have it. I put it in my purse when I got the call to come down here." Rifling through a badly frayed cloth purse, she pulled out a three-page document and handed it to Brooke.

As Brooke looked it over, Mrs. Reynolds said, "I pay that man Antonee $500, and he tells me if any one of my sons dies, and they donate their parts, I get $50,000 per boy. Like I said, life on the streets be mean, and I don't want to lose another son to those damn gangs. So, I signed the paper before Tayjon was killed. I need the money. You understand."

Brooke was scanning over all three pages, and what she was reading seemed to match precisely what Mrs. Reynolds was saying. The paper was an insurance policy, and the premium was a one-time cost of $500 for all the children Mrs. Reynolds had, and on the form was a listing of Tayjon, Ashari, and their brother, Jeffery. The policy was from a company called TTWC Insurance. It stipulated that if Mrs. Reynolds or any of her current living children or any other children in the future died and their organs were donated, she would receive $50,000 per child.

Also listed was a 1-800-(ARCHORG) number to call if her children were near death so the organs could be harvested properly. After the phone number, highlighted in bold type, was the statement: To receive payment, the donor must be transferred to the Arch City Transplant Center immediately upon death.

As Brooke was trying to process what she was reading, she looked out from the window in the office and saw Allison walking towards her with, she was sure, news about Ashari. News Brooke assumed was not good.

Allison walked in emotionless and knelt next to Mrs. Reynolds, but instead of telling her of the loss of yet another child, she said, "Mrs. Reynolds, good news. We removed the bullet from Ashari, and he went to the ICU. He is still very sick and weak, but we are hopeful."

"Praise the Lord, praise the Lord, praise Jesus," shouted Mrs. Reynolds with tears in her eyes. "Can I go see my boy?"

"Not yet, Mrs. Reynolds. He is being transported now, but let's give the team about 30 minutes to get him all settled in, and I will come back out to get you. Ok?" Allison answered while patting Mrs. Reynolds's hand.

"Ok. I wait," was all Mrs. Reynolds could muster as the stress zapped the air and energy from her body.

"Also, Mrs. Reynolds, the police need to talk with you because Ashari was shot. There was a boy who brought him in, and they will want to know who that was. They will be by in just a few minutes," Allison added.

"I don't want to talk to no police. They don't care about us. We do our justice on the street. We find who shot Ashari, and we even up the score," said Mrs. Reynolds, now defiant again.

Allison had heard this street justice bullshit before, so she cut Mrs. Reynolds off immediately. "Be that as it may, Mrs. Reynolds, you must talk to the police. What you say, how much you help them is your decision, but I can tell you, I wash blood out of my uniform every night, the blood of the innocent and the guilty, all serving their form of street justice. I am glad that Ashari is stable. But this bloodshed must stop, and maybe telling the police what you know will help. But that is your decision."

Once Allison left the room, Mrs. Reynolds turned to Brooke and said, "Damn right, it is my decision."

Trying to change the subject as Brooke was unsure if Mrs. Reynolds would bolt before the cops showed, Brooke brought Mrs. Reynolds back to the policy. "Mrs. Reynolds, would you mind if I took a photo of your policy just in case we need it for anything in the future?"

Mrs. Reynolds looked at Brooke warily but said nothing, so Brooke took out her phone and took a few photos of the policy, then handed it back to Mrs. Reynolds. "Let's hope you never have to cash in this policy," Brooke said, but Brooke was not sure Mrs. Reynolds had the same sentiment.

They both turned towards the door as a plain clothes Detective appeared, handing her card to Mrs. Reynolds and introducing herself. "Mrs. Reynolds, I am Detective Rhonda Simon, and I am here to ask you some questions about your son's shooting. Ashari, correct? That is his name?"

Mrs. Reynolds looked at the card and just nodded. Detective Simon had seen this act before. Pure hatred of the police department. Turning to Brooke, Detective Simon also handed her a card. Brooke reached to shake Rhonda's hand and said, "Nice to meet you, Detective. I am Brooke MacIntosh, and I work at the hospital but not in E.R. I was just down here visiting my friend Dr. Quillen, and she asked me to help calm Mrs. Reynolds down while the team worked on her son."

"Ok, Ms. MacIntosh. If you have nothing pertinent regarding this situation to add, you can excuse yourself."

"No, nothing I can add here," said Brooke getting up from her chair, but as she did, she cast an eye towards Mrs. Reynolds and then back to Detective Simon, who picked up on the tell. Brooke wanted to speak to Detective Simon but did not want to do it in front of Mrs. Reynolds.

"By the way, where do you work at the hospital, Ms. MacIntosh?" Rhonda asked.

"I work up on five in the transplant unit. Got a few hours left on my shift, so I better get back up there," Brooke replied, giving Detective Simon the green light to follow up with her when she finished with Mrs. Reynolds. Brooke left, and Detective Simon turned her attention to Mrs. Reynolds and the mystery shooting of her son, Ashari. He was lucky, so far, not to be victim 106, 116, or 126 this summer. Rhonda was losing track, but she also knew that Ashari, if he survived and made his way back to the street, would eventually be a future victim or would be administering his justice for this shooting.

CHAPTER 46

Vinnie had four names on his list. Marvin Applebaum, Steve Darcy, Jonas Stecker, and Raul Montez. All of them were good matches for Frank, and maybe one of them was the perfect match. He was still unsure what he was supposed to do with this information, but the person who gave him the list told him that if he wanted to save Frank, one of these people on this list would be able to do it. Thinking an idea would come to him if he could meet or see these people, he decided to visit Marvin Applebaum in an assisted living center in Chesterfield, a suburb 20 miles west of St. Louis. Vinnie had never done anything like this, casing people, but being an avid reader and watcher of crime movies, he believed he had a basic understanding of the steps to follow. Entering "A Peaceful Gathering Place" Assisted Living Center, he walked up to the reception desk. He asked to speak to the manager, stating that he was considering putting his brother in a facility and wanted to get a tour. Vinnie had seen this simple request work every time in his crime novels, and sure enough, within a few minutes, a young woman named Sally appeared with the title on her nametag saying: Visitor Coordinator. After repeating the same story as he told the receptionist, Sally immediately began Vinnie's, aka Thomas Riley's, tour.

Sally walked Vinnie through all the common areas: the cafeteria, the exercise facility, the library. In every room, she pointed out the happy and fulfilled residents, who, to Vinnie, looked anything but fulfilled or happy. Sally took Vinnie down a hallway past open and closed resident rooms, telling him she would show him an empty room so as not to disturb any residents. Vinnie glanced at all the names on the doors. Most of which had photos of the resident as they looked today and in happier, younger times, along with smiling family members. They were probably smiling because they unburdened themselves by dumping their responsibility off at a nursing home.

Once shown the empty room, Vinnie asked pertinent questions about mealtime, activities, and amenities that could be brought into the room. Then, hoping to see more of the facility, Vinnie asked, "Are there any larger accommodations for my brother? Perhaps one with a small kitchen with separate sleeping and living rooms?"

After passing several apartments, Vinnie saw the name Marvin Applebaum on a door. He knew that Marvin Applebaum was only 70, so he hoped he was healthier and more independent and would be in a larger, more self-sufficient apartment.

Stopping and not asking Sally for permission, he knocked on the door and said to Sally, "Oh, Marvin Appelbaum is here. I need to say hi to him. He's an old friend of the family. He would be thrilled if my brother came here."

Before Sally could throw out any concern about following protocol, the door opened, and Marvin Appelbaum, 5'8" with silver thinning hair and dressed stylishly, appeared in front of Vinnie. Sally did not want to anger a potentially lucrative client, and she also knew an apartment like Marvin Appelbaum's was worth $10,000 a month to the facility. So, she didn't say a word.

"Can I help you?" he said in a voice stronger than Vinnie would have imagined.

"Hi, Marvin. I am Tom Riley. You may not remember me, but you were a friend of my brother, Roger Riley."

"Roger Riley? It doesn't sound familiar, but you know I have trouble remembering what I ate for breakfast, let alone people from my past." Vinnie knew because he spent a career in sales that the best way for someone to open up is to find common ground, and the best way to find common ground was to see something in their office or home that you could instantly bond with over. Vinnie then glanced at some photos on Marvin's door and noticed one in front of the Missouri Botanical Garden.

"Roger worked at the Botanical Garden, and I know you, and he talked about all the wonderful gardens there," Vinnie said.

"I love the Botanical Garden. Does Roger still work there?"

"No, not anymore. Roger is retired, and we need to move him into an assisted living place. He's been suffering from dementia for quite some time. Do you still get to the gardens anymore, Marvin? Roger would love to go, but it's more and more difficult for him to go by himself."

"Oh, I hope he does move here! It is such a nice place with nice people, and we go to the garden every Wednesday at 10:00 in the morning. He should join us one day. I would love to see him again," replied Marvin.

Knowing he had pushed this ruse as far as he could, Vinnie said his goodbyes to Marvin, and then acting as if he had run out of time, he bid Sally a hasty goodbye and told her he would set up a time for his brother to visit the facility in the next couple of weeks. Leaving the assisted living facility mentally exhausted yet full of himself for pulling off the charade he had just performed, Vinnie decided the next person to see on his list was Steve Darcy, who lived about four miles east in Town and Country.

Vinnie drove east and entered the neighborhood where Steve Darcy lived. Luckily for Vinnie, the homes in Steve Darcy's neighborhood, sitting on one-acre lots and worth several million dollars each, were not protected by gated street entrances, as the crime was low in Town and Country. Vinnie turned right on Topping Road, then left on Old Colony Lane, and looked at house numbers featured on each of the elaborate brick-encased mailboxes lining the street. Finding the address, Vinnie pulled his truck behind some landscapers working on the neighbor's home. He hoped Steve Darcy or any other neighbors would not notice him, as his truck could be mistaken as a landscaper's. While Vinnie waited, he pulled up LinkedIn and Facebook to see if he could find more information about Steve Darcy. Both social media sites supplied ample information, both personally and professionally. It seemed Steve Darcy owned a very successful marketing agency in town that serviced various clients in the marine and RV industries. Based on the company's website and listing of employees, Vinnie assumed at least 100 employees worked for Steve Darcy. On Facebook, Vinnie could determine that Steve Darcy and his family were outdoor enthusiasts, probably related to his business focus. Many photos and posts showed Steve Darcy and his family enjoying many outdoor pursuits. Based on the pictures, Vinnie figured out that Steve Darcy and his wife had three children that looked to be between 8-15 years old. As Vinnie perused the Facebook posts, he heard a beeping horn, and a Black Cadillac Escalade pulled into the Darcy driveway, towing a beautiful Nautique wakeboard boat. After a few more horn beeps, the front door opened and what looked like the entire Darcy clan, including a Golden Retriever, bolted out of the house to meet their father, Steve Darcy. Based on the children's excitement and attention toward the boat, Vinnie guessed the boat was a new addition to the Darcy family. Vinnie marveled at some people's success and wealth at a young age. Steve Darcy could not have been more than 40 years old, maybe 45, and in front of his multimillion-dollar home, he also had a Cadillac Escalade and premium boat that together had to be worth at least several hundred thousand dollars. Yes, Steve Darcy was living the American dream, and making matters worse, Steve Darcy looked like a golden boy. He also looked a little taller than Vinnie, with an athletic build accentuated by his fashionable clothing. He and his family looked like they all could be models for an Orvis magazine ad.

As Vinnie looked at the scene in the driveway, he wondered why Steve Darcy was on the list of perfect matches for Frank. He was young and looked like the picture of health. Did Steve Darcy have some sort of terminal illness? Perhaps that is why he bought this new boat. Maybe Darcy knew he was dying. Vinnie hoped that was not the case and that Steve Darcy was not a future perfect match, as he knew death to Steve Darcy would have long-term devastating effects on the Darcy family. As Steve Darcy and his family continued to gawk over the boat, Vinnie took a photo of Steve with his phone in case he needed to meet with him again. Not wanting to press his luck, Vinnie started his truck and drove off. It was now nearly 4:00 p.m., and Vinnie was tired. He decided to wait until tomorrow to check out the other two match candidates: Jonas Stecker and Raul Montez.

CHAPTER 47

Detective Simon had finished interviewing Mrs. Reynolds to see if she could shed any light on her son's shooting. She couldn't. Mrs. Reynolds did not know the name of the boy Ashari was with, but the boy seemed to know her well enough to call when Ashari was shot. She did not know the names of any of Ashari's friends. She did not know where Ashari was early in the day. All she knew was that Ashari was a good boy, "never in no trouble," according to Mrs. Reynolds. Rhonda told Mrs. Reynolds to call her if she remembered anything or if she heard anything about who might be the shooter. Rhonda knew she would not be receiving a call. However, before Mrs. Reynolds got up to leave, Rhonda remembered a case not too long ago.

Reynolds? Reynolds? Detective Simon thought. She said, "Ma'am, did you have a son named Tayjon Reynolds?"

"Yes, I did. And you did nothing to lock up the drug dealers who killed him with that poison," Mrs. Reynolds replied.

When Mrs. Reynolds left, Rhonda noticed that the business card she handed Mrs. Reynolds earlier was left lying on the table. After Mrs. Reynolds left to see Ashari in ICU, Rhonda sat down, sighed in weary exasperation, and thought, *if this kid's mother doesn't seem to care about solving this case, why the hell should I?* Gathering herself, Rhonda went to the elevator and pressed the button for the 5th floor, where she hoped Brooke MacIntosh had some insight into this crime.

Upon getting off on the fifth floor, Rhonda went to the nursing station to ask for Brooke. The nurse at the desk told Rhonda that Brooke was making rounds, but she would text her to let her know Rhonda was waiting. Rhonda did not need to flash her badge as she did not want Brooke seen as someone talking to the cops. After a few minutes, Brooke came around the corner and greeted Rhonda warmly. "Detective Simon, hi. I didn't realize you would be here so soon." Brooke had no concern that others might see her talking to a detective, and as Rhonda glanced around, she could see no one was paying attention to them as the nurses and doctors were very busy dealing with their issues.

Brooke pointed down the hall and said, "Let's go to the employee lounge. We can talk there." As they walked to the employee lounge, Rhonda could tell that Brooke commanded respect and attention as she saw it in the eyes of her co-workers who nodded and smiled as she passed. Quickly sizing up Brooke MacIntosh, Rhonda assumed she was going somewhere in her career and life. Sitting at a table strewn with a mixture of old fashion entertainment and medical magazines, Brooke cleared them off, and the two women sat down.

Dog-tired, Detective Simon got down to business immediately. She asked, "Brooke, I sensed you wanted to talk with me but not in front of Mrs. Reynolds. Is that correct?"

"Yes, Detective, it is. I wanted to speak with you about something that may or may not have anything to do with the shooting of Mrs. Reynolds's son. I wanted to tell you in private because it may involve Mrs. Reynolds and possibly be related to two other recent murder victims."

With that, Rhonda became more attentive. "Ok, Brooke, you have my attention."

"Well, when I talked to Mrs. Reynolds, she mentioned something about her having an insurance policy on her son that would pay off $50,000 if her son were to die."

"So," Rhonda replied, "many people have insurance policies."

"True," Brooke said, "But she also mentioned the policy was activated if her son, or any of her sons for that matter, died and donated their organs, which I thought was odd."

"Odd, how so? I am not an expert on insurance policies, but I know some of them have riders or clauses for special circumstances. Could the organ requirement be something like that?"

"Maybe, I guess," Brooke said, "but let me run something else by you." Detective Simon was quiet, so Brooke continued. "Well, as you may or may not know, it is illegal in the United States for people to receive compensation for donating an organ. I think the only country that allows it is Iran. However, some countries have very active black markets where I am sure the selling of organs takes place."

Intrigued and thinking about Tayjon Reynolds, the methhead whose kidney was cut out, Rhonda asked, "Do you know of any such activity in the states?"

"No, not really, and not in any transplant operations I have ever heard about, but who knows what happens on the dark web?"

Rhonda knew about the dark web. It was where all the scary shit, with dangerous people lived, breathed, and plied their illegal trade, supposedly hidden from law enforcement, but Rhonda knew the FBI, CIA, and NSA were all secretly infiltrating the dark web.

"Ok, what else about Mrs. Reynolds' insurance policy caused you some suspicion?" Rhonda asked.

"Mrs. Reynolds was not the first person to mention this in the ER. Over the last several weeks, two other mothers of murder victims both mentioned this policy and the need to collect $50,000. My friend, Dr. Allison Quillen, who works in the ER, told me about those cases, and that was why I was down there today. Allison texted me when she heard Mrs. Reynolds mention the policy."

"Well, I may need to talk to Dr. Quillen, but if this is a case of insurance fraud, that is not my area of responsibility. Those are usually federal matters. However, if they connect to the shootings, I will chase them down."

"That's the thing, Detective, I think it may be both," said Brooke.

"How so?" asked Rhonda.

"I think, maybe, and I know this sounds crazy, but maybe the victims are being killed specifically for the harvesting of their organs."

Detective Simon's first reaction, which she kept to herself, was that Brooke MacIntosh was reading too many medical science fiction novels. Still, in the short time she had known Brooke Macintosh, she sensed that she was a serious woman, not prone to wild thoughts or conspiracies. Plus, Rhonda did not think her theory was that off base. It could happen. People are murdered for no reason, for every reason, and for some reasons you don't want to imagine.

Finally, Detective Simon said, "Brooke, this sounds intriguing, and I will follow up with Dr. Quillen, but unfortunately, I have my hands full with solving five other murders. Plus, the two victims you mentioned who came through the ER with those policies are not my cases, but I will check with the Detective handling those.

Closing her notepad, Detective Simon got up, weary of the onslaught of murder and unsolved cases. She liked her murder cases clean. Drug deals that went bad, lovers quarrel, or gang retaliation. Organ selling and complex insurance fraud linkage were not what she needed at this point.

"Well, if there is nothing else, Brooke, I will be on my way. I may run back down to the ER to see if Dr. Quillen is still on shift."

"Ok. I know the insurance fraud angle is not really what you do, but do you want to see the policy?" Brooke asked Detective Simon.

"You have it?" Rhonda asked.

"Yes. Mrs. Reynolds let me take some photos of the policy on her sons," Brooke said as she showed Rhonda the policy photos on her phone. Rhonda swiped through three screens before stopping at the policy's issuer: TTWC Insurance Company.

Brooke, knowing what Rhonda was looking at, said, "TTWC. I was going to look them up online but got busy once I got back on my floor. Probably some initials of the company founders from 100 years ago."

"No, Brooke. TTWC means "Their Time Will Come."

"That's a creepy name," Brooke said. "How did you know that is what those initials meant?"

"Because I met the President of the company two days ago. If you would, can you text me these photos? I will try and find Dr. Quillen, but if you see her first, please tell her not to mention these policies to anyone.

And Brooke, the same goes for you. Do not look up this company online and don't have any digital interaction with them that could link back to you. Go back to your job and let me handle things from here."

"Am I in danger, Detective?" Brooke asked, suddenly scared for the first time in her adult life.

"You are in no danger if you follow my advice but call me if you hear of any other policies floating around or hear of anything that might be related to this company."

Detective Simon got up, and Brooke walked her to the elevator. The strong, confident woman Detective Simon saw in Brooke just 30 minutes ago was replaced by a scared young woman wondering what she might have stumbled into. What Rhonda did not know about Brooke was that while she may be temporarily frightened, she was not paralyzed by fear and planned to investigate TTWC as she needed to learn how they and the Transplant Center were connected.

CHAPTER 48

Vinnie returned to his home after researching two of the four potential donors he had selected. As he contemplated what to do next, he decided to check in on Frank to see how he was doing. He decided to call versus text as he felt he needed a real conversation to evaluate Frank's mental state and condition better. Calling his cell phone, Frank's wife Sue answered instead of Frank.

Immediately in Sue's voice, Vinnie could tell she was down. Usually an upbeat person, regardless of the circumstances, Sue's voice now seemed weary, tired, and deflated.

"Vinnie, I'm so glad you called."

"Is everything ok? You sound down. How is Frank?"

"I am ok, I guess. Frank is sleeping. We just got back from his rehab at Barnes, and he just wanted to go to bed when he got back. I am getting more and more worried about him every day."

"Sue, that is understandable. Frank is very sick, and he knows it, but when I have been with him, he seems to be committed to rehab and getting ready for a transplant. And he will get a transplant. I just know it."

Sue countered, "I am not so sure about that. Every day we wait either someone else has gotten a transplant or someone we got to know at rehab has died because they did not match soon enough. Frank is beginning to think that no matter how hard he works to get in shape, he will run out of time and luck."

Vinnie didn't know what to say, so he said nothing.

Sue broke the silence and said, "I just don't know what to do if Frank dies. He is the rock of this family. Frank's positive outlook always kept my spirits up even in the toughest periods of our marriage and life."

"How long do you and the doctors think Frank has before he needs the transplant?" Vinnie asked.

"Well, the doctors are kind of vague about it. They keep encouraging him to work hard, and they will be ready when he is ready. They are more positive than us about finding a match for him."

"What about you? What do you think?" Vinnie asked Sue.

"I think weeks. I think Frank has weeks to find a transplant, not months. We have agreed to take any donor that matches him. He would be better off with the lungs of a lifelong smoker than his lungs at this point. By waving all the donor restrictions, we had hoped we would move to the top of the list, but that has not happened. That is why he and I are starting to face the reality that he may not get the lungs he needs."

"Sue, I didn't want to get your hopes up, so I did not tell you, but I asked Ellen to see if there is anything she could do because of her work at the Transplant Center."

"And?" Sue said with a bit more enthusiasm in her voice, "Is she able to help?"

Vinnie did not know how to answer Sue's question as he was sure the donor list he now possessed came, if not directly, indirectly, from Ellen and the Transplant Center. He also knew that acknowledging the list would create more questions from Frank and Sue about what Vinnie planned to do with the information. Plus, the man who gave Vinnie the list threatened Vinnie with physical harm if Vinnie shared acknowledgment of the list with anyone.

"No, unfortunately, she can't do much," Vinnie told Sue. "I think she talked to Frank's doctor about his case, but organ donation is so strictly controlled by the government that there is not much they can do for Frank."

"Well, thanks for asking her, and tell her we appreciate her trying to help. I think it is in God's hands now whether Frank lives or dies," Sue said.

Vinnie was not a believer in divine intervention. He was only a believer in taking matters into his own hands, and in Frank's case, Vinnie was wondering how to do just that.

Testing the water to see what Sue's reaction would be, Vinnie asked, "Would you or Frank ever do something illegal or unethical to get lungs for Frank?"

Sue's answer was quick and expected. "No. We put our faith in God. If Frank getting lungs is part of God's plan, he will get them; if it is not, we will accept that fate." She added, "You know, Vinnie, you sound a lot like our boys who read this stuff on the dark web about black market organ donors."

"Yeah, that is kind of why I asked the question. I hear there is a market for this, mostly overseas, but I guess someone in the U.S. is doing this. If there is a way to make a buck, you have to figure someone is willing to commit a crime to do it."

"I think people are making more than a buck, and from what our boys tell us, illegally obtained organs cost hundreds of thousands of dollars. While we would do anything we could for Frank, we would not commit a crime, and of course, we don't have any money to do something like that. Although it could mean Frank living, I know Frank could not live with himself if he did anything like that."

Trying to sound a bit more cheerful as he ended the call, Vinnie said, "I know, I know, just playing my usual 'what if' with you. Tell Frank I am thinking about him and please call me if you need anything or anything changes with Frank. And tell him I called and will try to come to visit in the next week or so."

"I will, Vinnie, and thanks for calling, but if you are coming for a visit, don't wait too long, if you know what I mean."

Vinnie hung up, exactly knowing what she meant, and he knew he would be visiting Jonas Stecker and Raul Montez tomorrow.

CHAPTER 49

Detective Simon went back down to the ER to see if Dr. Quillen was still on shift, but she had already done her 12 hours and was at home. Rhonda knew the hours these ER doctors put in, so she did not want to wake Dr. Quillen at home, so she would visit her when she was back at the ER. Besides, Rhonda was chasing down the connection of the murder victims in the carjacking cases that were more important to her than the most recent gunshot and stabbing victims from the ER.

Using case.net, Missouri's online database for court cases, she quickly researched all the cases Kim DeAngelo may have worked on during the five years she spent as a lawyer in the St. Louis prosecutor's office. Not wanting to eliminate any possible cases, Detective Simon downloaded a summary of all cases during those five years. She planned to show these cases to a former employee of Bill Thomson's high-end PI firm, SCOPE. Simon felt it would be easy for a case name or two to ring a bell with the SCOPE contact. She printed off the list and headed to meet Richard Leary, one of the original employees of SCOPE, a former military running mate and lifelong friend of Bill Thomson. When Rhonda talked to him on the phone, Richard Leary was more than willing to help solve the murder of his best friend, regardless of if he was under a SCOPE NDA.

They agreed to meet at Helen Fitzgerald's located in Sunset Hills in south St. Louis County, a very popular watering hole for the avid sports fans of St. Louis. Since the meeting was scheduled for mid-afternoon at 3:00, Rhonda assumed the place would be a little quieter, but she was wrong. Helens was bustling with customers enjoying 28 screens of live sports from any part of the globe, cold beer, and perhaps most importantly, air conditioning on a typically 90/90/90 summer day in St. Louis, with 90 degrees, 90% humidity, and 90% chance of rain. Rhonda also noticed that half-price beers and well drinks started at 3:00, not the typical 5:00 p.m. happy hour, as this place catered to the blue-collar construction workers who began their day at 6:00 a.m. and got off work and started drinking at 3:00 p.m. Moving through the crowd, Rhonda made it to the back booth of the bar, where Richard Leary waited in what Rhonda assumed was his bar domain where he could keep an eye on the crowd. Richard Leary was ex-military. Not only had he kept habits from his military and investigative days, but he was also, while over 65, still showing hardened facial features and a very chiseled body, with sinewy muscular forearms, probably from hours of intense workouts every morning. His grip when Rhonda shook his hand was vice-like. Richard Leary was one badass dude, not to be called an old-timer, and Rhonda guessed most people in the bar steered well away from him.

He motioned Rhonda to sit down, and when he smiled, he showed perfectly white teeth, not the yellow-stained teeth most people of his age seemed to have. His voice was gravelly and deep, not from smoking, she guessed but trained from quiet conversations he probably had in bars like this around the world.

"I drink bourbon, and I don't take you for a Chardonnay kind of woman, so what will you have?" he asked Rhonda, not caring she was still on duty as he knew Detectives lived by their own code. Rhonda also knew how to get someone to talk, so she was willing to drink with them.

"Bourbon is good. Neat. Woodford Reserve will do."

Nodding in approval, he held up his hand with two fingers raised to signal the bartender across the room. Rhonda immediately liked Richard Leary. He was the type of man she wished she found herself with more often, but she seemed to end up with the poorer, cruder version. Although

Rhonda felt that Richard Leary could have five more drinks and his mind would still be sharp, she needed him lucid. Wanting to get into the list sooner than later, Rhonda immediately pulled out the casc.nct list.

Looking down at the listing of all the cases, Richard laughed out loud, saying, "Detective, if we are going to go over all those cases, we will be here awhile. I'll order some food. The grub here is pretty damn good."

Rhonda did not resist and let him order, which he did without even looking at the menu. For her part, Rhonda did not make an excuse that she was tight on time. *Maybe Richard Leary,* she thought, *would serve some value more than confirming a few shared cases.*

Taking the list from Rhonda, he started running his finger down each case, reading the brief description of the case and the plaintiffs. He then said, "I look at this list of cases, and I wonder about the future of humanity. Don't' you, Detective?"

Rhonda, of course, had the same thoughts every day but just responded, "Mr. Leary, I know this is a lot to go through, so I appreciate you doing this."

He put his hand up to stop her. "Detective, If I can help find that son of a bitch that killed my friend, I will stay all night doing it. And call me Richard."

After 20 minutes of looking at each case, interrupted by another round of drinks and delivery of some chicken wings and Kobe beef sliders, Richard Leary pulled out a pen and began circling a few cases. As he did, he would scroll through his phone, looking at corresponding emails that helped him confirm his recollection of the cases. Finally, after 45 minutes, he reviewed all the cases and handed the list back to Rhonda.

"Detective, the ones I circled are cases that SCOPE also worked on. I am 100% sure of these. As you can see from my notes, I recall some others, but I can't ascertain whether we worked on them or sounded familiar because they were in the news. I hope this is helpful."

Rhonda looked at the list. Richard Leary had circled three cases, none of which had any meaning to Rhonda, so she asked Richard if he recalled the nature of the investigations SCOPE performed on the cases.

"As you know, Detective, SCOPE investigations specialize in tracking the digital footprints of white-collar criminals. Mostly bad actors working for and usually ripping off the companies they work for.

In most cases, SCOPE was tracking embezzlement or money laundering. You know, financial stuff. In our cases, clients hired us to investigate a suspicion they had about a crime committed by one of their employees. These first two cases, if I recall, were simple money embezzlement cases where internal company accountants were setting up a payment to fake vendors that never existed. Pretty typical white-collar crime, usually done by the most unassuming man or woman in the office."

"Ok, what about the third one? St. Louis City was pursuing a case against Life Health Clinic?" Rhonda asked.

"That was an interesting one, but it was primarily Bill's case as it dealt with selling illegal drugs, and Bill had a hard spot for anyone who sold drugs since his oldest son died of opioid addiction. Two doctors owned life Health Clinic. I can't recall their names, but we assisted the St. Louis prosecutor's office directly in investigating this operation. One of the doctors was writing opioid scripts to an unsavory group of people who then would sell the drugs on the street. If I recall correctly, this became a big operation, maybe the biggest supplier of prescription drugs in the city for a while, and this doctor was raking in the coin, big time. But he was dealing with some scary people moving this shit. He would be caught by us or capped by his street boys. Lucky the law got to him first. Probably saved his life."

While Rhonda knew she could probably pick up the investigative thread on the case using police resources, she wanted to push Richard Leary a little harder for two reasons. One, because she felt he had more information to give, and two, because she was hoping Richard Leary could be more than a one-time information source. Rhonda slid over slightly closer to Richard, giving him, she hoped, a signal that she wanted more information, or maybe she just wanted more of him. "Richard, is there any more information you can get me on the doctor and who the prosecuting attorney was on the case?"

Richard patted Rhonda on the hand and told her to wait as he had to get something out of his car. A few minutes later, Richard returned with his laptop and opened it up.

"It is easier to look this up on my laptop than on my phone. Fat fingers, you know," he said.

Punching the keyboard for a minute, Richard went through a series of computer commands before he got the screen he wanted. Sensing Rhonda wondered about all the extra steps he took, Richard answered her, saying, "We are on a public network, and the information I am pulling up is best left hidden from hackers. So I am using my encryption codes to get into a back door of SCOPE's database." He then turned to Rhonda and said with an amused grin, "Now, Detective, because this information is so sensitive, I will need to only give it to you verbally or send it to your personal email. So, if you can write that down, and maybe your phone number, you know, just in case I have other information I need to give to you at a moment's notice, I would greatly appreciate that."

Rhonda laughed and wrote her email and phone number on the back of her card. Sliding it over to Richard, she said, "Just don't do any of your digital trackings on me, Mr. Leary. All you'll find is that I lead a boring life, work, work, work. No play, and certainly no excitement to speak of recently."

Not taking his eyes off Rhonda, he said, "Yep. That describes my life, as well." He wrote a few lines on a napkin and then handed it to Rhonda. He said, "Maybe this will help solve the case you are working on, so perhaps you will get some more free time in the future."

On the napkin were words that would probably keep Rhonda very busy for the short term but would help free her up in the future.

Prosecuting Attorney: Kim DeAngelo, Defendant: Dr. Kenneth Thorton, CEO of Life Health Clinic

Looking up from the note, Rhonda turned to Richard Leary and asked, "Richard, you said two doctors owned the Clinic. Who was the other one?"

After entering a few more commands into the database, he turned to her and said, "Dr. Alex Finnegan was the other owner."

"Thank you, Richard. I think you have helped a lot and while this may add to my workload in the short term, let's toast to some free time, fun, and excitement in my future." Clinking his glass to hers, he added, "our future."

CHAPTER 50

Vinnie got up, knowing he had a full day ahead for scoping out both Raul Montez and Jonas Stecker, and after his conversation last night with Sue, he was beginning to feel that time was of the essence. Based on the addresses he was given, both Montez and Stecker lived in apartment complexes in St. Louis. He would check out Raul Montez, who lived just west of Forest Park on Wydown Blvd, a nice area and street west of Washington and Fontbonne Universities and populated with young urban professionals, college students, and college professors. Based on some internet research, Vinnie determined that Raul Montez was a professor of Architectural Design at Washington University, and perhaps the best time to see him was in the morning on his way to class.

Jonas Stecker's apartment was in the Soulard area, which was much less affluent than where Montez lived, but Soulard was a popular place for young, single people and creatives.

Based on Vinnie's research Jonas Stecker spent his days working as a bartender at Hammerstone's, a restaurant in Soulard. However, Stecker was primarily an aspiring saxophonist and played many gigs with a band called Brothers Roosevelt around town. If he missed Stecker in the morning, and he assumed based on his choice of professions, the morning hours did not agree with Stecker, but he would easily be able to track him down at the restaurant or one of his band's gigs.

Going first to Raul Montez's apartment, Vinnie parked on Wydown within 30 yards of Montez's building. It was a well-kept, two-story, gray brick building and, by the looks of it, had four apartments. These apartments usually were rented to professionals or academics as the rent would run around $2500 a month, high enough to keep out the underemployed but not so high that it created a constant turnover. The street was very busy with walkers, joggers, and parents taking their kids to the school bus stop. It was a charming neighborhood, with low crime and access to the universities to the east and the Clayton business and entertainment district to the west.

Vinnie had a picture of Raul Montez that he downloaded from the internet on Washington University's academic staff page. He sat for 20 minutes, and as luck would have it, Raul Montez exited his building with a bike in hand, and as he put on his helmet and secured his pants leg, he hopped on the bike and rode east. Vinnie assumed he was heading to his job at Wash U.

Vinnie followed behind him in his car. Raul rode his bike through Brentmoor Park, a desirable neighborhood of stately old homes. Raul then turned right onto Forsythe Avenue, going east and towards Wash U's main campus. Knowing he would not be able to follow him easily in the car if he got on campus, Vinnie saw a sign for a public parking garage. After traversing several levels, Vinnie pulled to the first open visitor spot he saw.

Vinnie didn't bother tracking down where Montez parked his bike. He knew it would be easy to find out where a professor of Architectural Design would be holding classes.

As he took the stairs from the parking garage to the campus, he looked at a directory and located the school of Architecture. He walked to the building, hoping to see Raul Montez entering, but he did not. Waiting until a few students strolled up to the front doors, he casually asked them if they knew what classroom professor Montez was lecturing in. Without any hesitation, they directed him to lecture hall 301. Feeling a kick of adrenaline, Vinnie bounded up the stairs to the third level and casually entered the lecture hall at the balcony level. Vinnie loved the feeling of a college campus and the freedom and optimism the students felt. College was a time when you believed you could accomplish anything. As Vinnie sat and listened to Raul Montez's lecture, Vinnie realized he had not felt unbridled optimism in a long, long time. Since his divorce from Ellen, it seemed that Vinnie had not accomplished anything and was just going through the motions.

Outwardly he portrayed joy and happiness, but something was dead inside him since the divorce. As he listened to the professor and scanned the bright students absorbing the information, he knew they had an un-limited future. Vinnie began to despair that he had no future, but that was because of his own doing. He then thought about Frank, who had no future, but due to nothing he had done. Vinnie knew the answer for Frank and maybe even himself, but he was afraid of what that answer might cause him to do.

Vinnie had heard enough of the lecture to get a feel for Raul Montez as a person. He was intelligent, though that did not matter much, and he looked in good shape and healthy. Again, like Steve Darcy, Vinnie wondered why Raul Montez was on his list. Looking at his watch, it was around 11:00, and Vinnie was hungry, so he decided to go to Hammer-stone's to see if he would be lucky and find Jonas Stecker working the lunch shift.

CHAPTER 51

With the information Richard Leary gave Rhonda, she now could make a connection with two recent murder victims. Bill Thomson and Kim DeAngelo worked on the same case, the case of former Dr. Kenneth Thorton writing illegal opioid scripts and using a network of drug dealers, selling the opioids on the street. All three of them crossed paths six years ago, but the question was: did they cross paths more recently when both Thomson and DeAngelo were murdered similarly at locations only a few miles apart and around the same time? Approximately 8:00–8:30 p.m.? Kim DeAngelo's killers were on camera, three young black men hiding in the garage stairwell before trying to steal her car and then killing her. In Thomson's case, a killing occurred, but the car was not stolen, probably because of the presence of Thomson's 6-year-old grandson. Rhonda did not have enough evidence to arrest Kenny Thorton. As for now, she could not connect him to those crimes. But after talking to nurse Brooke MacIntosh about the mysterious insurance policies owned, ironically, by mothers of young black men, she had an excellent reason to talk to Thorton again.

Detective Simon arrived at Kenny Thorton's unkempt house. Knowing that Kenny was involved and found guilty in the criminal act of selling opioids, Rhonda wondered why he was living here and not in state prison. But how was he paying for his house since he got out of prison? His car? His lifestyle?

Perhaps his role as President of TTWC Insurance was legit and paid him handsomely, but all that would come out in time. Rhonda hoped this unannounced visit would be the unraveling of whatever bullshit story Kenny Thorton was about to lay on her.

She rang the doorbell and waited. Just like her last visit, it took a few more rings for Kenny to finally appear from within the house to greet her at the front door.

"Detective Simon, how nice to see you again, and so soon. Did you just drop by because you are in the neighborhood, or is this an official visit?"

"How about we call it a social visit? A chat between two friends," Rhonda replied.

"Fair enough, Kenny said, "and if it is anything more than a nice chat, I probably would ask my lawyer to sit in."

"If it is anything more than a social visit, we would be doing this down at the station. I assure you, Mr. Thorton."

"Fire away, Detective. I am all ears."

Rhonda, noticing Kenny was certainly less friendly on this visit, jumped right in, "Ok. Your insurance company: TTWC. Who would you say is your typical customer?"

"Anyone looking for low-cost insurance to insure their most valuable assets, themselves and their family."

"So, no type of demographic or racial focus? Let's say selling policies to underserved members of society, like black, Hispanic, immigrant families?"

"That, Detective, is discrimination and, of course, illegal. So, no. We sell policies to whoever needs them. Do you need a policy, Detective?" Kenny replied.

"No, I am good. Covered by the police union. I am curious as to how the policy pays off?"

"Well, each policy is different, but in most life insurance policies, payment is made upon a person's death."

"Are there any other criteria required for policies? I think they are called riders to a policy?" Detective Simon asked.

"Sure, many policies have riders that increase or decrease the cost of the policy. You know, like smoking or risky lifestyles. For example, Detective, you would have a higher premium because you are in a dangerous job that could get you killed."

Rhonda wondered for a moment if that was a veiled threat. She then asked, "What about requirements that a policy only pays if the person covered donates their organs."

With a bit more enthusiasm, as if he was proud of that fact, Kenny answered, "Internally, we call that our "Pay It Forward" policy. It is an ingenious concept I came up with to encourage more people to become organ donors. The policy pays off more and is less expensive if someone is willing to donate their organs. You may or may not know, Detective, but organ donation is a real problem today, especially with the minorities of this country. In a small way, our policies are trying to improve that by encouraging more organ donations. I am very proud of what we are doing in this field."

Surprisingly, Rhonda thought the "Pay It Forward" concept sounded like a good idea but pushed Kenny a bit more. "So, you don't consider the "Pay It Forward" concept a way to get around the illegality of paying someone for their organs?"

"No, and you know what else, Detective? Neither do regulators, as all we do is encourage organ donations as a requirement for the policy to be paid off. No one is putting a gun at these people's heads to donate their organs." Rhonda found Kenny's choice of words a bit ironic.

Kenny continued, "I must say, Detective, last week you sat on my porch and asked me about my car's involvement in potential carjackings or murders, and this week you are asking me about insurance policies. Do you have a specific point you are trying to make or is it a slow day, and you are chasing conspiracies?"

Ignoring Kenny's question, Rhonda pressed on to see how far Kenny would go before lawyering up.

"Kenny, what is your relationship to Arch City Transplant Center?"

"They are a client of ours. Many who are about to die or have died are transported there for the eventual process of organ donation. No different than a family asking the hospital to transport their loved one to a specific mortuary upon death."

"Do you have any other clients like this?"

"If I did, I would not tell you as I have confidentially agreements with my clients, like any business would, Detective."

Sensing that Kenny may get tired of this cat and mouse game very soon, Rhonda changed course, seeing what time of reaction she would get from him. She could tell he was a very intelligent person as he handled each of her questions with not a bit of stress or guile. "Kenny, can you tell me about the time in your life when you were a doctor and owned Life Health Clinic?"

Kenny just sat back and smiled. Rhonda knew the cat and mouse game was about to end.

"Well, congratulations, Detective. I am glad you learned to use Google to research me, or was it case.net? It doesn't matter either way. You know all about my time at Life Health Clinic. I was a doctor. I sold opioids. I got arrested and convicted, served my time, and am now making amends to society and trying to improve my life. Is that now a crime, Detective?"

Rhonda got up from her chair, knowing the conversation was at its stopping point. Based on the information Brooke told her, Rhonda decided to press Kenny and said, "It's not a crime turning your life around, but how you may be turning your life around may be a crime. Over the last several weeks, several young black men have come into the Barnes ER shot or stabbed, and all of them had relatives, probably their mamas, claiming they were to be paid off by TTWC for their organs if they got them to The Center. Tell me something, Kenny. You seem to be buttering both sides of the bread, Kenny. Maybe selling the policies, ensuring they get paid off by causing the death of an insured person, then Arch City and your buddy Finnegan prosper by getting the organs."

Kenny quietly looked at Detective Simon, then smiled before laughing out loud. "Detective, before I tell you to get the fuck off my porch, I have to compliment you for trying to tie me into every single crime committed in St. Louis in the last month. It must help your closing rate if you can wrap up all your murders with one suspect. I guess it gives you more time to shoot some innocent black guy for a speeding ticket. Before I call my lawyer for harassment, are there any other crimes you want to accuse me of doing? If not, get the fuck off my porch."

As Rhonda got back in her car, she knew she had pushed Kenny Thorton as far as she could without charging him with a crime, but she needed more pieces of the puzzle to fit before that could happen. He was right in that it seemed she was all over the place, chasing his involvement from carjackings and murder and now following up on a possible pay-for-play organ/insurance scams. Rhonda was beginning to feel the investigation tentacles were expanding beyond her reach, but she knew someone who might be able to help. Pulling out the napkin from the night before with his number, she took out her phone and texted Richard Leary: "Care to do nice cop a big favor?" Immediately, he responded: "Deal, and when done, I look forward to how you may pay me back."

Chapter 52

Vinnie pulled up a stool at Hammerstone's, and after ordering a beer, he looked over the lunch menu. Vinnie ordered what his doctor told him not to eat: a burger and fries. While he waited, he sat listening to the intermittent conversation between the two bartenders as they waited on customers. He hoped he would pick up on the name Jonas Stecker without asking, as Vinnie did not want himself identified as being in contact with Stecker. Within a few minutes, he got the break he was looking for as one of the bartenders yelled out, "Jonas, can you grab me a case of Bud Light? This cooler is almost empty."

Jonas Stecker did not seem pleased to handle the request as he grunted and said, "Sure, Brittany, I can do your job and mine," adding "bitch", muttered under his breath as he headed out of the bar area. Moments later, he returned with a Bud Light case and set it down near the cooler below the bar. He gruffly asked, "I guess I have to put them in the cooler, too?" Brittany, who seemed to be the more senior of the two, answered bluntly, "Yeah, Jonas. I got my fucking hands full over here, so pull the stick out of your ass and help."

Vinnie always preferred sitting at a bar while eating alone as he loved interacting with the bartenders and the customers. He always felt the vibe of any restaurant was better witnessed at the bar, as employees and customers felt freer to talk among themselves. He was counting on this because once Jonas was busy at the far end of the bar, he asked Brittany, "Man, what's the deal with that guy? Is he always so surly?"

"Yeah. He's an asshole most of the time. He only helps at the bar occasionally when his band has a gig here at night. Frankly, I think the guy is homeless because he always hangs out here when he is not working."

Vinnie said, "Well, I hope he is a better musician than a bartender."

Brittany laughed, "Not much better. The band he plays in is pretty good, Brothers Roosevelt, and Jonas isn't a bad sax player, but he is no Charlie Parker."

"I am impressed, a young woman like yourself brings up Charlie Parker. Not really your generation."

"Mister, jazz lives in all generations, and Charlie was and will always be the best in my book."

"Your friend Jonas surprises me. Most musicians, especially sax guys, are mellow. I guess Jonas is not that way."

Brittany answered, "Jonas, mellow? Hell no. It's like he's always got a hot poker up his ass. He seems to hate everyone, hates life, hates himself. Probably because he has served some serious time down in the Potosi state pen. I can't stand working with him, but he only works here a few hours every other day, so I chill by putting on the buds and tuning him out."

Vinnie didn't want Brittany to sense he was probing too much about Jonas, so he changed the subject. Vinnie pointed to another beer and said, "Well, I hope your playlist includes some good Kamasi Washington."

Brittany just smiled, maybe flirting a little with Vinnie. "If any dude can pull out Kamasi for a playlist, you are worth buying a beer," she said as she poured him a fresh one. Feeling a little flattered and taken aback, Vinnie thanked Brittany for the beer and promised to come by some time to check out the music, but he planned to focus only on one person in the band: Jonas Stecker.

CHAPTER 53

For two reasons, Richard Leary was anxious to work on the project Detective Rhonda Simon had told him about. First, he had not done much digital snooping since he left SCOPE, and he missed it. Plus, if what he did could help solve Bill Thomson's murder, he was all in. He knew the cops had their hands full with exploding crime rates and reduced staff and budgets, not to mention the growing chorus of Defund the Police, which limited budgets. Anything he could do to back the blue, he would. His second reason was more personal. Detective Simon was the type of woman he was instantly attracted to. To him, confident, brash, and tough traits increased her sex appeal and allure. It had been a while since Richard had been seriously involved with a woman, and he was hoping Detective Simon would be more than a professional relationship.

What she asked him to do might take some time, but he still had all the software necessary to find out what Detective Simon was after. She wanted Richard to go back as far as needed to determine the complete history of the business and personal relationship between Kenny Thorton and Alex Finnegan.

The most challenging decision was to determine how far back to go. Since they were doctors, he figured medical school time frames would be a good starting point as medical schools have limited alumni, so the search there would be very concentrated.

His results came up quickly and easily since both Kenny Thorton and Alex Finnegan went to Washington University Medical School at the same time. Then he looked at residency programs. Though Thorton did his residency in Miami while Finnegan went to Chicago, Richard wondered if Thorton began using drugs and turning to criminal ventures in the Miami drug and crime-fueled culture.

After residency in the early 2000s for Thorton and Finnegan, they returned to St. Louis. Finnegan worked full-time for Barnes Hospital, while Thorton worked for St. Louis University Hospital.

After a few years at Barnes, Finnegan took an unexpected turn, leaving medicine temporarily and getting his MBA from Northwestern University. *Intelligent and brave guy*, Richard thought. He was leaving a lucrative profession and getting an advanced business degree at a top university. Finnegan was a man with a plan. Thorton took a less steady path, leaving life in the hospital and starting his own business, Life Health Clinic, which he started around 2010. At this time, Finnegan finished his MBA, did a stint with a Private Equity Firm in Chicago, then returned to St. Louis and reunited with Thorton at Life Health Clinic. Richard did not know what it took to start a clinic, but he figured big bucks. So, perhaps that was the expertise and contribution Finnegan brought back from the financial sector.

This time frame would be where Richard Leary would get the most private information. While digital snooping has been around since the digital age began in the mid-90s, the proliferation of every social media platform, legit and non-legit, exploded in the 2000s, as did digital snooping tools, web crawlers, social media scraping tools, and illegal hacking techniques.

Richard Leary could and would use all tools at his disposal. Scraping all the social media contacts, conversations, photo sharing, etc., would be time-consuming but easier than hacking into Finnegan and Thorton's email, phone, and text records while at Life Health Clinic. It would take some time, but Richard Leary was a motivated man.

After several hours of snooping, Richard Leary texted Rhonda, indicating he had some interesting information to share. He suggested they meet somewhere less public than a restaurant or bar, and when she suggested he come over to her place, he readily agreed.

Richard planned to show up at Rhonda's around 7:00 p.m. Sensing and wanting the evening to extend beyond a work discussion, Rhonda changed into her best-fitting jeans and an off-the-shoulder black ribbed blouse. She decided the best course of action was to settle business first and then see how the night progressed. Leary rang her bell precisely on time. Leary dressed casually in knee-length khaki shorts, an untucked floral shirt, and black sandals. His skin bronzed, and she could see his legs were as muscular as she noticed his arms were the first night they met. He had a laptop bag over his shoulder, so Rhonda assumed he was all business tonight. He extended his hand for a greeting, making Rhonda glad they didn't fall into the hug versus handshake awkwardness professional males and females seemed to find themselves. She directed him to her kitchen table, where he laid down his bag and opened it to pull out his laptop. But also handed her a bottle of Buffalo Trace Bourbon, saying, "My mother told me never to enter a friend's home empty-handed," adding, "but let's wait till I show you what I have found before you open that."

It would be business first, then maybe pleasure, Rhonda thought.

"Detective, do you want the data unfiltered and straight at you or the full explanation of how I found what I am about to show you?" Leary asked.

"Well, I don't want you to reveal any of your trade secrets because if any are illegal, I might have to arrest you," Rhonda laughed. "So, just the straight dope, so to speak."

Winking at Rhonda, Leary said, "Ok, let's avoid the arrest and handcuffs for now and get down to it. Some of these folks were and still are up to no good."

Leary did a quick summary of his research in the early academic and professional years of Drs. Finnegan and Thorton. He started his in-depth investigation when the two became business partners. "What we have is Finnegan and Thorton, old med school buddies, in business together at Life Health Center. I believe Finnegan to be the money man behind the business. After a few years of a very profitable and growing business, the shit starts to hit the fan as Thorton seems to be involved in an opioid venture that is bringing lots of unreportable cash to him, and perhaps to Finnegan, as well. And as you know from public records, Thorton was brought to trial and convicted of selling prescription opioids on the street."

"Ok, Richard. So far, I knew most of that, though, I did not realize Finnegan and Thorton knew each other so far back."

"Patience, my dear, patience, and you will be rewarded with some fine sipping whisky when done here."

"Now, through my unique talents and the software I own, I dug deeper and discovered that Finnegan perhaps knew more about the opioid scheme than he ever let on. I think he was the brains of the operation, but he let or persuaded Thorton to be the fall guy as Thorton had a drug problem well before he started the clinic. You see, Finnegan is a long-term, big picture guy, and he was laying out his Arch City Transplant plan years ago, and a drug conviction would have squashed this potential billion-dollar score."

"Do you have proof that Finnegan let Thorton take the fall?" Rhonda asked.

"Would email correspondence between Finnegan and Thorton be proof enough, Detective Simon?"

Rhonda nodded, not asking nor wanting to know where Richard Leary got the email proof. She simply said, "Go on."

"Ok. So now we bring it back to public records. We know that Kim DeAngelo, the prosecuting attorney, worked with SCOPE and Bill Thomson specifically to get the dirt on Thorton and Finnegan, and they had them dead to right. It was an easy white-collar conviction, but a missing piece of the puzzle to me, and I am sure to the prosecuting attorney, was who was moving the opioids through the streets of St. Louis? Thorton or Finnegan was not on the street corners selling this stuff. So, who was their distribution contact?"

"Hold that thought for a minute, Rhonda," Leary said. "You would think it would be a big win and feather in the DA's office connecting white-collar criminals to the inner-city drug problem, and it would score some points with the boys in City Hall," Leary continued.

"Yes, I would think so. Why are you about to tell me I am wrong?"

"Patience, my dear. Patience. All good things happen slowly," he winked at Rhonda. The guy moving the opioids on the street was an easy find. You may even know this guy. William Burroughs."

Rhonda sounded surprised when Leary mentioned the name. "William Burroughs was moving the opioids on the street for Thorton and maybe Finnegan?" she asked.

"So, you know him?" Leary said.

"Well, about two months ago, I was scraping his brains off the wall in a home in north city," Rhonda replied.

"Well, a few years before his splattered brains met your acquaintance, he turned state witness for his part in the opioid trafficking. He made a deal with the DA for a reduced sentence which was quite an ask for a guy going into the joint for the 4th time in his 10-year crime career."

"So, he turns on Thorton and Finnegan in exchange for reduced time?" asked Rhonda.

"Only Thorton. It seems Finnegan cut a deal with the DA that had him set up both Thorton and Burroughs in exchange for his immunity. As I said, Finnegan is a long-haul thinker, and even back then, he was a mover and shaker in this city in the medical, business, and charitable fields. He has backers with deep pockets, which also help elect some local politicians, many of whom might benefit from riding the Finnegan money train in the future. Plus, the DA had Burroughs looking at a long, long stretch at Potosi correctional. So, once Finnegan fingered him as the local distributor, it was an easy take for Big Willie to turn evidence on Thorton in exchange for a reduced sentence."

Rhonda asked, "Ok. That makes sense that Finnegan, to save his hide, flips Burroughs to the DA, but why would Finnegan turn on Thorton, his longtime friend and business partner, and why now, if he did turn on Thorton, would Thorton still maintain a business relationship with Finnegan?"

Leary replied, "Finnegan is a visionary and brilliant businessman, but one who sees legitimacy in business as a complement to criminal activity. He also plays the game for the long haul. Based on reading between the lines of Finnegan and Thorton's email correspondence, there was a two-part plan. First, he convinced Thorton that Burroughs flipped on Thorton of his own volition to get a reduced prison sentence. Then Finnegan told Thorton that he was doing everything possible to help Thorton get a reduced sentence. Finnegan promised Thorton a steady income stream while in the joint and most assuredly when he was released. Finnegan convinced Thorton that he would lose his medical license as a known drug user, so only getting an extra year for drug trafficking as a reduced sentence deal was a gift to Thorton that Finnegan brokered."

Rhonda added, "Thorton must be a little gullible to believe Alex Finnegan was helping him."

"Maybe more than gullible. Thorton and Finnegan were extremely tight. Finnegan was the alpha dog, top of the pack in med school, and Thorton just idolized him and thought he could do no wrong. In Thorton's mind, it was noble to take a bullet for Finnegan so they could benefit in the future. Thorton knew that Finnegan was the star of their operation. And I believe Finnegan held to his promises to Thorton because as odd as it seemed, despite all the success and adulation Finnegan receives, I think Kenny Thorton is Finnegan's only true friend," Leary explained.

Rhonda asked, "Besides the Transplant Center, being a customer of Thorton's insurance company, TTWC, do you know if there is any other connection between the two entities?"

Laughing, Richard Leary said, "Alex Finnegan may think he is smarter than the rest of us, but I found out what he is up to. I have digitally tracked the movements of foreign leaders, mercenaries, drug lords, and arms dealers worldwide. And, when I entered private practice, some of the most ingenious white-collar criminals and I would place Alex Finnegan on the pantheon of ingenuity based on how he set up TTWC."

"What do you mean?" asked Rhonda.

"Alex Finnegan knew that Kenny Thorton, as a convicted opioid drug dealer, would not be looked favorably upon if he was to apply for a license to own a life insurance company. So, Alex Finnegan, a medical and business star, applied and got the license. But as he formed the company, Alex hid the true ownership under an offshore corporation, whose sole owner is, in fact, Kenny Thorton."

"Why would Finnegan set up Thorton as the owner?" Rhonda asked.

"My guess is because if TTWC engages in illegal activities to benefit, perhaps indirectly, The Transplant Center, no roads lead back to Finnegan. They only lead back to Thorton, who unfortunately will again be the fall guy for Finnegan if all of this comes crashing down."

Rhonda said nothing for a while as she thought about all that Richard Leary had uncovered.

She began to feel sorry for Kenny Thorton that he was such a pawn for Finnegan, who indeed was an evil puppeteer pulling Kenny Thorton's strings, but did he pull them enough to cause Kenny Thorton to murder him?

"Richard, this is a lot to think about, but you have certainly earned your reward for the night," she said as she walked over to the bourbon and poured two glasses.

Clinking his glass to Rhonda's, Richard Leary smiled and said, "I hope this isn't my only reward tonight." Leaning over to light two candles on the table and dimming the overhead lights, Rhonda kissed Richard and whispered into Richard's ear that perhaps he should plan to spend the night.

CHAPTER 54

A fter her enjoyable evening and morning with Richard Leary, Detective Simon thought that the best course of action was to squeeze Kenny Thorton tighter and give him an updated history lesson on the whereabouts of three individuals: William Burroughs, Kim DeAngelo, and Bill Thomson, all killed, and all connected to Kenny's past life at Life Health Clinic. While it would be easy to connect Kenny with the revenge killing of all three of these individuals, as they certainly impacted Kenny's imprisonment, Rhonda still did not believe Kenny had murderer DNA. However, the more she learned about Alex Finnegan, the more she thought he possessed the evil, hidden darkness, ego, and narcissism most murderers had.

Detective Simon thought about how she wanted to squeeze Kenny. She was unsure what leverage she had on him to make him cooperate as she could not connect him directly to the murders. All she had was a connection to the victims from years past. She had two choices. One, the old school approach of following Thorton on his daily routine, and two, the high-tech way: get Richard Leary to follow him digitally.

She decided for the time being to go old school and see if some good old-fashioned police work would uncover something that would make Kenny Thorton more talkative. She also had a card or two in her pocket based on information Richard Leary had turned up about TTWC and its true owner. Information Rhonda believed would open Kenny Thorton's eyes about being played the fool by Alex Finnegan once again.

Based on her previous meeting with Thorton, Rhonda knew he was not necessarily an early riser, so she headed to his house around 9:00 a.m. to see when he might start his day.

As she suspected, his white Audi was in the driveway. So, he was still home, probably still in his bathrobe sipping coffee. Thirty minutes later, Thorton merged from his house, started his car, and headed east towards downtown. Rhonda followed him, thinking he was perhaps heading for his office, if he had one, though she suspected he was not a 9-5 office guy. As he got into the downtown corridor, he took a left on Broadway and headed north past the underused convention center, the Dome at America's Center, the former home to the St. Louis Rams football team. He stayed on Broadway for several miles before turning west towards the entrance of Bellefontaine Cemetery. Rhonda thought it was odd that Kenny Thorton would visit the old cemetery, but perhaps he had a relative buried here and was paying his respects. She suspected Thorton would not recognize her car, but to be sure, she waited across the street from the entrance, assuming Thorton, if visiting a relative, would drive directly to the grave site. However, he stopped at the visitor building immediately inside the gate, where he exited his car and began walking to his destination. Rhonda turned into the entrance and parked about 50 yards from where Kenny had parked, but she could see him take a road over a small hill.

She hurried to the front of the Visitor's Center to ensure she would not lose sight of him, and being unfamiliar with the many paths and roads of the cemetery, she grabbed a map. While she was in this general area many times investigating cases, she never came into the cemetery. While it was historic and beautiful, it gave her the chills. All cemeteries did. Bounding up the same hill that Thorton had crossed a minute earlier, Rhonda was glad to see not only was he still in view about 100 yards ahead, but she also had ample places to conceal herself as she could duck behind large monuments, obelisks, or oak trees.

Rhonda looked at her map, which not only pointed out the many roads but also pointed out the many significant grave sites. Based on her map and the direction Thorton was traveling, he was headed to a large monument, signifying the grave of William Clark, the slightly lesser known of the Lewis and Clark exploration team. Rhonda moved to Kenny's left, still about 100 yards away, where she had a clear view of the well-manicured and final resting place of William Clark, whose centerpiece was a 35-foot granite Obelisk. She was surprised by two things as she sat and watched. First, the cemetery in the daylight was beautiful. Massive monuments to the dead surrounded by lush gardens, large trees, and placed or planted flowers. Secondly, she was surprised that Kenny Thorton's reason for being here was not to pay respects to the dead but perhaps to pay respects to those who caused death. Waiting for him at the grave site were the three young males Rhonda was pretty damn sure were the same men on video carjacking and killing Kim DeAngelo. She was too far away to hear what they were saying, but she could see them hand several documents to Kenny. In turn, Kenny handed over what seemed to be a significant amount of cash. A financial transaction was taking place, maybe drug-based, but perhaps more information-based, due to the presence of the documents. She waited, hoping that a gun would not appear, and she would need to expose herself, with no backup to stop a crime. After a few minutes, the meeting ended amicably as Kenny and the one man doing all the talking slapped hands, and then each left in different directions. The men headed north on foot, presumably back to their stomping grounds, and Kenny headed back towards his car.

Rhonda dashed and darted between the trees and monuments as she wanted to reach Kenny before he got into his car. As he approached his car and reached for his keys, Rhonda came up behind him, surprising him by saying, "Interesting friends you keep, Kenny."

Kenny turned to Rhonda with a smirk. "Oh, Detective, I wish I knew you were here. I would have introduced you."

"No need to, Kenny. I think I already know who they are. They are those nice young lads that jacked and then killed Kim DeAngelo, aren't they?"

With his smirk now wiped off his face, Kenny showed a bit more concern than in any past conversations he had with Rhonda. "How do you know that? How can you be so sure?"

"I am not 100% sure, Kenny, but I bet if I dragged your smug ass down to the station and showed you the video, you would 100% agree with me."

"Listen, I know these guys aren't angels, but I don't think they are killers," Kenny said with more doubt than he was conveying. "They are trying to make a go of it legally," he added.

"How so, Kenny? The papers they handed you for the wad of cash you gave them certainly looked suspicious. You want to tell me about that?"

Kenny said, "Listen, Detective. I don't have to cooperate with you at all as I know my rights, but I am because my dealing with these guys is legit, and I have nothing to hide." Kenny pulled the papers and handed them to Rhonda. "Look, this is what they handed me, sold insurance policies for my insurance company TTWC."

Rhonda took her time to look at all the paperwork; they seemed like legitimate insurance policies. The policies were like those that Brooke MacIntosh shared with Rhonda a few days ago.

"Ok, Thorton. These seem to be legit policies, but what's with the meeting here in the cemetery, and why cash? It doesn't smell legit to me."

"Detective, you know the streets. You know how hard it is to break away from the gangs and go straight. For these guys to do their job, they need to keep their actions off the grid. That is why I meet them here in private so that they can get in and out unnoticed. And you know the reason I pay in cash? Because real money is the only currency that the streets respect, besides guns and drugs. I pay them cash when they sell each policy, and they can use the cash to recruit new guys for me or spread the money around any way they choose."

Rhonda thought for a while. She was going into an area that was close enough to arrest Kenny now, at a minimum, for accessory to murder. Still, he was cooperating, and she wanted to get more information from him, either to charge him, squeeze him or maybe uncover something bigger. "Ok, Kenny. Let's say you are legit with these guys, but here is where you are in deep shit. I'm pretty sure these hoodlums are the guys who capped Kim DeAngelo, and my guess is they also killed Bill Thomson and William Burroughs. I assume all these names should ring a bell for you, Kenny."

Kenny said nothing, thinking perhaps about the names or maybe buying time to wiggle out of this.

"How do you know they are connected to all these murders?" Kenny asked seriously.

"Good police work, Kenny. And you know what else? Good police work will have you connected to them, and in case you are not in a talking mood, let me help you connect the dots."

"No need, Detective. I will do it for you. William Burroughs sold my opioids on the street. Then he turned on me for a lighter sentence. Thomson investigated me, and DeAngelo tried me. I can add a few more names to the Kenny Thorton shit show, which is how I describe my past if you have any other unsolved murders, but I think these will suffice for now."

Rhonda was surprised Kenny was so forthcoming and had to decide right now if it was time to arrest Kenny and read him his rights, but she sensed that if she hauled him in, he would immediately lawyer up.

"Listen. You are close to reading my rights and arresting me, so if that is your move, go ahead, but before you do, let me say one thing. There is not a Kenny Thorton shit show revenge tour. I have moved on and am trying to make amends for my life. If all these crimes are connected, you know they are not random killings as I am connected to all the victims. It should be an open and shut case. So, here are my wrists. Cuff me, Detective. However, before you do, and while it looks bad for me, the real question you and I are both thinking about right now is, who is behind the killings? Because you know these guys, whether they did all three or not, are not acting on their own."

Rhonda nodded her head, indicating she was thinking along the same lines. "So, how do we find that out, Kenny?"

"You make sure I am legally protected and, most importantly, physically protected from revenge from these guys, and I will find out who is behind it. It would be much easier for me to get this information while working on the street, instead of in the can, don't you think, Detective?"

"I think you should follow me to the station of your own volition, and let's get you what you need." With that, they both got into their cars. Kenny followed Rhonda out of the cemetery to the precinct a few miles down the road.

CHAPTER 55

Detective Simon and Kenny Thorton met in her office at the precinct. As they drove down separately, Rhonda felt her original read on Kenny Thorton was the correct one. This guy may have led a shit show of life, as he so aptly described, but a killer did not seem to fit his personality. Plus, he seemed so forthcoming in their conversation at the cemetery that he had to be telling the truth about his lack of involvement with the DeAngelo, Burroughs, and Thomson killings.

Grabbing a small office to afford some privacy, Rhonda offered Kenny a cup of coffee, "Kenny, I can grab a cup of coffee for you, but I have to tell you it's about 3 hours old and not as tasty as what you gave me at your house the other day."

"Water is fine, Detective," he replied.

After handing him a water bottle, Rhonda wasted no time setting up what she hoped would happen here. "Kenny, I want to record this session, so there is no confusion about what we discussed. Is that ok with you?"

"Yep."

She pressed the record button on her phone and placed it between her and Kenny. "First, I want to identify myself as Detective Rhonda Simon, and I am speaking with Mr. Kenneth Thorton. Mr. Thorton has come into the office of his choosing. I have not placed Mr. Thorton under arrest nor given him his Miranda rights, though he knows he can request them anytime. He also is aware that if he chooses to have a lawyer present, he can. Is that correct, Mr. Thorton?"

"All good and accurate, Detective. Let's get this show on the road," Kenny said rather enthusiastically.

Rhonda decided to give Kenny the information in stages and see his reaction. She still needed to see if any part of what she was telling him surprised, angered, or encouraged him to add some of the missing pieces. She also knew that if Kenny was involved in the killings, her approach was risky as a good lawyer could probably get any charges dropped relatively quickly based on Rhonda's approach. She first went through the opioid conviction of Kenny at Life Health Clinic using general searchable information. She left out the details that Richard Leary, who she did not identify, had discovered about Alex Finnegan's role in the events. This was information in which she wanted to get Kenny Thorton's reaction, and she assumed it would be a strong one.

"Kenny, have I accurately described your role in all of this? The trial, conviction, etc.?" she asked.

"Yep. You hit all the highlights of the low lights of my life," he said solemnly.

"Ok. Kenny, William Burroughs, who was peddling your opioids on the street, turned against you. His testimony primarily convicted you, but do you know how turning William Burroughs came to be?"

"I guess the DA squeezed him pretty hard, and he did it to reduce his sentence. Not sure why as it seemed he spent most of his time between ages 16 and 25 in prison, so what's a few more years to a loser like him?"

Rhonda countered, "Big difference spending 15 more years or two years, and that was a compelling offer to make Burroughs talk."

"Probably, I guess," replied Kenny, head down, seemingly uninterested in reliving the past. "I am glad he won't spend more time in jail wasting our taxpayer money."

"Ok, Kenny. Now let me share some information that I have gotten. First, we know that Alex Finnegan, who you go way back with, was deeper in this opioid deal than came out in public, and we know that he convinced you to take the fall."

"Yeah, he said I was going to lose my medical license anyway because of my drug use, and if I took the rap, he would make sure to take care of me. A year in prison was tough, but he did take care of me, kept up the payments on my house so I wouldn't lose it, and set me up once I got out. Prison sucked, but I guess that's behind me now." Kenny said this without anger, without remorse, almost confirming that he was not on some revenge tour.

"Ok, what if I told you that it was Alex Finnegan who flipped William Burroughs to the cops. Does that surprise you?"

Kenny smiled a bit at Rhonda and said, "Nothing Alex does ever surprises me, but I just thought that was good police work, Detective, finding Burroughs as my street connection as he was a well-known dealer at the time." Thinking a bit more, Kenny added, "I guess the thing that does surprise me a little bit is that Alex took the chance naming this guy, knowing that Burroughs's people would have no problem finding and killing Alex."

"Well, I think that Burroughs got a great outcome with a reduced prison time, but I guess Finnegan probably ensured that Burroughs's gang still had supplies to move on the street. Keep the money flowing, and everyone is happy, right Kenny?"

"Alex always knew how to take care of everyone and wrap everything up tightly. He has a gift," was the only thing Kenny added.

"Yeah, he's special," Rhonda said sarcastically. "He has a gift for making big money and having influential friends all over this city. And you know what influential friends like better than money? They like no loose ends."

"What do you mean?"

"Your friend Alex Finnegan is about to make it big time. Not big, like a wealthy guy in St. Louis who has a luxury box for the Cardinals and shows up on society pages, but big, like one of the richest men in the country if his plans for Arch City Transplant achieve what he and his investors hope it will. Guys like Alex Finnegan, guys like his investors, plan for everything, and if anything might be a problem, they eliminate it."

"I am not following, Detective," Kenny said.

"You, Kenny, are the problem. You are a loose end. And from what I can tell, you may be the only loose end left who knows something about Finnegan's role in Life Health Center. You see, Kenny, all the loose ends are gone. William Burroughs, the snitch, is gone. Bill Thomson, the investigator, is gone. Kim DeAngelo, the prosecutor, is gone. Maybe there are a few more we don't know about, but all the big trails leading to Alex Finnegan are gone. Except you."

"But I am still here. Alex is taking care of me. Hell, he appointed me President of his insurance company. He is helping me turn my life around. You got it all wrong about Alex."

"Well, regarding the insurance company, Alex Finnegan did something nice for you. Thanks to some corporate manipulation Alex Finnegan performed, you are not just the President; you are 100% the owner of TTWC."

Looking confused, Kenny said, "I don't understand. Why would he do that and not tell me?"

"Because when TTWC serves its purpose of finding more donors to The Center, it and you are expendable. Finnegan is a guy that always pushes the boundaries of what is legal and ethical, and while TTWC may be useful to Finnegan today, my guess is once Finnegan no longer needs TTWC, he will close shop on it and you. He won't risk the billion-dollar potential of the Transplant Center to protect TTWC or you. And by the way, my friend, his backers, who are big donors to politicians and probably to the insurance industry, have the leverage for TTWC to get shut down and for you to earn a lifetime stint at a maximum-security prison. That is your next home when Alex Finnegan decides you have served your purpose."

"That makes no sense. Alex knows TTWC helps those underserved by giving them financial security if their loved ones die, plus it becomes a source of future donors. He told me so," Kenny added, sounding exasperated on hearing all of this.

"Speaking of future donors, do you think Alex Finnegan has any involvement in those who are insured being killed?" Rhonda pressed ahead.

"Wow, even for Alex, that seems like a reach. Alex does not and would not facilitate the killings. He set up TTWC assuming, rightfully so, that many insured people will die eventually based on street violence and revenge justice. I can't believe he would get his hands so dirty as to accelerate the killings," Kenny said.

"Maybe you are right, so let's leave that for now. Kenny, I know you mentioned you pay off; what do you call them, your agents, in cash, right? How do you get paid?"

"Cash," Kenny responded.

"And how do any policies get paid off?"

"Cash. I do it myself because it is a lot of money," Kenny answered.

"Kenny, you are a smart guy, smart enough to know it is unusual for a business to pay off claims and employees in cash, correct?"

"Alex never wanted the paper trail because he..." Kenny stopped in mid-sentence. He looked directly at Rhonda, who answered, "So he does not have a paper trail to lead back to him, right Kenny?"

"That mother fucker. He is setting me up again."

Rhonda nodded. "It would seem so, but more importantly to you right now, could he possibly be setting you up for the murders of DeAngelo, Thomson, and Burroughs? You may spend some time in a minimum-security prison for any insurance fraud TTWC may be charged with, but you will die by lethal injection if charged for murder."

"But why would he do that, Detective?"

"Loose ends, Kenny. Loose ends. Alex Finnegan is about to become a billionaire, and Alex Finnegan's investors and political backers are about to become richer and more powerful. You, Kenny, are the last loose end that connects Alex Finnegan to his past that DeAngelo, Thomson, and Burroughs knew about."

Kenny went pale. All his detached and laidback attitude was now gone. Rhonda could tell he was scared, so she gave him some hope.

"Kenny, let me tell you how I think we can turn this around on Finnegan, save your hide, and who knows, maybe even make TTWC a legitimate business you can be proud of."

Once done explaining her plan, Kenny nodded in agreement and said, "Alex took my life away from me once. I won't let him do that again."

Chapter 56

Vinnie decided to check in on Frank this morning before he went to the Club to play golf and have lunch.

Dialing Frank, Vinnie was hopeful of good news.

"Hey, Frank. How are you doing this morning?"

Frank answered quietly in a weak voice, "Always good to be upright in the morning, Vinnie. I am good if I start and end the day that way."

"Any news on a lung donor?" Vinnie asked.

"No, no news on that front. Always trying to be hopeful, but it's tough to be positive when it seems my clock is ticking down. To be honest with you, Vinnie, if I don't get lungs, I hope to go quickly and not cause any more pain to Sue and the kids."

"Frank, don't talk like that. I know you will get them, and I think it will be very soon. I can feel it."

"Well, one way or another, Vinnie, I think the end is near. I hope not, but it seems this is just not going to go my way."

"Just hold on, Frank. Hold on. Good luck is just around the corner. I will call you tomorrow, but if you get any news on the lung, call or text me. God bless, Frank." Vinnie hung up, more anxious for Frank than ever.

Vinnie felt guilty that he had good health and was out enjoying an afternoon golfing while his brother-in-law was weeks away from death. After his call with Frank, he left to play golf, but his round was not satisfying as he couldn't get his mind off Frank and his condition. It was not unusual for Vinnie to have a drink after golf. However, what was unusual even for him was that by 2:00 p.m., he was shit-faced drunk, turning from happy-go-lucky to belligerent.

His mood was turning dark and dour as he debated whether to try driving home or call an Uber. Unfortunately, he soon crossed paths with the one person that would make his mood worse than it was, Alex Finnegan, who had arrived at the men's grill in advance of an afternoon game. Finnegan and Vinnie usually ran in different circles and played golf at different times, so any chance encounters were minimal or during large events. Today was one of those encounters. With some liquid courage and vile coursing through his veins, Vinnie yelled over to Alex, sitting a few tables away, "How are we so fortunate to have Dr. Death come down from his throne to grace us with his presence?"

Alex ignored him, sensing immediately Vinnie was drunk and any confrontation would escalate.

Being ignored, Vinnie yelled again, "Hey Finnegan, you think you can play God, but how come you can't help my brother-in-law, you ass-hole."

Again, Finnegan refused to take the bait and decided the best course of action would be to move out to the course and leave Vinnie to focus his ire elsewhere. But Vinnie followed him outside and berated him as he walked towards the Pro Shop. Now worried that Vinnie would cause an uglier scene than Alex or the Club would tolerate, he turned back towards Vinnie and said, "Let's not make a scene you are sure to regret," and grabbed his arm and threw him in a golf cart, driving them both off quickly to a distant corner of the course. Vinnie, while protesting, was too drunk to stop Alex and knew better than to try and jump out of the cart.

Stopping behind a maintenance building and out of view of anyone, Alex turned his anger on Vinnie.

"Ok, Calabrese. I get that you are drunk and angry because of your brother-in-law, but I have no problem giving you a serious beat down and leaving your sorry ass out here. Is that what you want?"

Drunk or sober, Vinnie knew he would not win a physical confrontation with Finnegan, so he just said, "No, what I want is you to help my brother-in-law. I want him to get lungs, and you can do it."

"I did what I could, Calabrese, but now it's in your hands," Alex said.

"What do you mean in my hands? What are you talking about?" said Vinnie, slurring.

"You have the names of four donors who would be perfect matches for your brother-in-law, and you have had it for weeks now."

"Wait, what? Did you give me that? I thought Ellen made that happen?"

'No, she did not, and you know the warning you got if you told anyone you have it. One tap on my phone, and you will get a visit from an associate of mine who will give you more than a beatdown."

"Why would you give me the list? Why would you help me?" Vinnie asked.

"I did it for Ellen, but what you do with it is your decision. But based on your brother-in-law's medical condition, I wouldn't wait too long to do something. He only has a few weeks left based on my evaluation."

They both sat in the cart, unspeaking. Finally, Alex broke the silence and said, "All those people on that list will die soon as they are terminal or have chosen the dignified way out through physician-assisted suicide, but the question is: will they die soon enough to help your brother-in-law? You may have the power to make that happen, but if you can't or won't, you're just a pathetic loser, but if you do, maybe you will save your brother-in-law and get Ellen back. Now get the fuck out of my cart."

Alex pushed Vinnie out of the cart and drove off. He hoped Vinnie would remember the conversation when he sobered up, but more importantly, he would do something about it. Alex had manipulated a smart guy like Kenny for many years, and he thought he could easily play a drunken dunce like Vinnie for the fool, especially using Ellen as bait. For love or money, Alex thought. He was counting on the depravity of human nature to better his agenda.

CHAPTER 57

After her interview with Kenny Thorton, Rhonda felt she was close to being able to solve the murders of Thomson, DeAngelo, and Burroughs, either individually or together, if they were connected as she thought they were. According to the information she had obtained from Richard Leary, all three murder victims were connected to Kenny Thorton and Alex Finnegan. They were all involved, either through the investigation, the finger-pointing, or the trial and conviction of Kenny Thorton for his opioid selling. Kenny Thorton had the most apparent motive if he was the killer of all three. Revenge. Get even. Payback. What bothered Rhonda was her gut told her Kenny Thorton did not seem like a killer. He seemed like a druggie in the past and maybe the present, but he was pretty laid back. He did not seem like a guy angry with a score to settle. He seemed like a guy who admitted his mistakes but was trying hard to turn his life around. He was very forthcoming in the interview and willing to work with her, which could be a deflection. Still, her experience told her she might be onto something bigger, something planned by a more prominent player, and that player might be Alex Finnegan.

She was unsure she had enough evidence to bring Finnegan in for questioning. Because she knew he was very connected politically, she had to have a rock-solid reason to do that, and all she had were assumptions of a motive, which frankly seemed flimsy. She needed collaboration from someone closely involved with Finnegan, and she thought interviewing and pressuring Dr. Ellen Calabrese may be a route she should take. She also thought she might be able to use Brooke MacIntosh, if she was willing, to trap Finnegan.

She knew neither Kenny Thorton nor Alex Finnegan pulled the trigger in any of the three murders. It was clear on video that three young black men killed Kim DeAngelo, and Detective Simon was 80% sure it was the same three men who killed Bill Thomson. And while there were no witnesses to William Burroughs's murder, Rhonda knew from experience it was done by someone in the neighborhood that most of the witnesses knew, and by knowing them, knew what the killers would do to them if they squealed. She also had the white Audi connected in some way to the suspects and the murders. She felt by arresting those involved with DeAngelo first, the other two murders would be easily pinned on them, as well, especially if they were willing to turn on their puppet master for a reduced sentence.

While she tried to stay focused strictly on the three murders, she was working on. She wondered if these three murders were in any way connected to the murders of the young men insured by the TTWC policies. Rhonda knew this was a stretch, but she had seen looser connections pan out in her work. There is a saying in the cops' and criminals' business that for the criminals to get away with their crimes, they must be lucky 100% all the time, and for the cops to catch them, they only need to be lucky once. Detective Simon needed a little luck and more reason to interview Dr. Calabrese. However, since she did not know her, she thought the best place to start was with Brooke Macintosh.

Dialing Brooke's number, Detective Simon was not sure of the reaction she would get asking Brooke to stick her neck in a case that a few days ago she told her to stay away from. When she left Brooke at the elevator banks, she saw fear but perhaps also saw determination.

"Hi, Brooke. Detective Simon here. How have you been?"

"Oh, hello, Detective. I have been good. Keeping busy with my patients but frankly still wondering about the conversation we had the other day about TTWC and The Center."

"It's interesting you are thinking about it because I have found out some more information that perhaps you may be of some help with."

"I am listening," Brooke said.

"First," said Rhonda, "I am sorry for scaring you when we met and warning you to stay away, but there may be some scary shit going on with some dangerous people both on the streets and perhaps connected to The Center and TTWC. I didn't want you to get involved and potentially get hurt."

"Well, Detective, I am already involved. I hadn't mentioned this before, but I have been meeting with Dr. Calabrese and Dr. Finnegan for the last several weeks, and they have offered me a job at The Center. To be honest with you, the meetings set off some of my internal alarms after and left me wondering who I may be getting into bed with."

"What kind of alarms?" Rhonda asked.

"Ethical, moral, legal. Their whole approach to changing the transplant business."

"Brooke, I am not a priest or a psychologist, so I don't get paid for solving moral or unethical dilemmas. I get paid for solving crimes. What is in your gut that makes you think they are doing that may be illegal?"

"Detective, you don't know me very well, but I assure you I am as steady as a rock and as reliable as the sun rising every day. When I tell you this, please don't think of me as a quack or millennial who watches too much TV. I am a very serious person."

"If I did not think of you as serious, I would have hung up five minutes ago. So, what has got you spooked?"

"The transplant business is all about supply and demand. The demand for people needing transplants is as high as ever, but the supply of donors never rises. I think Arch City Transplant and maybe this insurance company TTWC are somehow involved in creating more supply."

"When you say supply, you mean more donors, right?" Rhonda asked.

"Right. I think the future donors may be the kids who are shot, and while Arch City may not be pulling the trigger, they are the benefactors if they can get these kids' organs."

"Brooke, if you ever sour on nursing, you may make a good Detective. I was thinking along the same lines. It might be far-fetched, but I think it's worth you and I sitting down at the station tomorrow to talk about how you may be able to help us sniff this out."

CHAPTER 58

Brooke was planning to meet with Ellen to discuss the new job on Thursday at the Transplant Center offices, so she arranged to meet Detective Simon on Wednesday at her office. Arriving at the precinct, Brooke was escorted back to a private room where Detective Simon and two other people were waiting.

"Brooke, thanks for coming in. This is Belinda Stevens, our surveillance specialist, and our assistant district attorney, Andrea Bottini. We want to review what we are doing here and ensure you are comfortable with the arrangement."

"Nice to meet you both," Brooke said. "As I told Detective Simon, I am very comfortable helping you out. What questions do you have for me, Ms. Bottini?"

"I understand that Arch City has offered you a job. Is that correct?"

"Yes, I have but have not accepted yet. I am supposed to meet with Dr. Calabrese about it tomorrow. They gave me an employment contract and an NDA," she said as she pulled it out of her purse and handed it to the assistant DA, who spent a few minutes looking it over while all others in the room stared silently at their feet.

She handed it back to Brooke and said, "This is a pretty standard document designed to keep you from moving on to work for a competitive company or sharing any trade secrets. I have no problems with you signing it as anything we learned via the wire would hold up against this in a court of law if we brought this to trial."

Brooke turned to Rhonda, saying, "A wire? A trial? I want to help, but I am concerned about what may happen to me if Dr. Calabrese and Dr. Finnegan find out I was involved in getting them in trouble.

Rhonda replied, "Brooke, we in no way are doing anything that we think will endanger you. We just want you to talk to Dr. Calabrese, and based on what we hear her say on the wire, it will help me decide how I want to approach her, as a guilty accomplice or a helpful ally. Nothing you ask of her would be outside the normal questions a new hire asks. What we are asking you to do is strictly voluntary, and by doing this, you will not be held accountable for any possible crimes committed by Arch City Transplant if you decide to take the job. Are you in or out, Brooke? Your decision."

"Ok. I am in 100%," Brooke replied, adding, "I am committed to saving lives, and I thought the Transplant Center was as well, and since I am pretty sure no matter what Dr. Calabrese tells me, I won't be taking a job with them. I will help any way I can."

"Ok. Now that we are good to go, we are ready to show you how to wear and activate this wire," Rhonda said, turning to Belinda Stevens. Belinda came around the front of Brooke and brought out a small transmitting device about the size of a hearing aid. "It's best if it's clipped under your shirt. Your bra would be good," Belinda said as she handed the transmitter to Brooke.

Brooke unbuttoned her blouse, trying different locations to attach the device to her bra. Each time she tried a new spot, she rebuttoned her blouse and stood up, asking everyone if they could see any signs of it. Settling on a location that was both comfortable for Brooke and unnoticeable to an outside observer, Brooke sat down and asked how the device got activated.

Belinda answered, "Brooke, we will text you a link to your phone. When you want to activate the device, just click the link, and it will activate from our end. When you want to deactivate the device, click it again." With that, Brooke's phone pinged, indicating an incoming text, and as she looked at it, she noticed it was from the "Food to You" company, which seemed to be a name for a food delivery service.

"Food to You?" Brooke asked quizzically.

Belinda answered, "Yeah, I know it seems stupid, but it is our internal name. It keeps prying eyes from seeing and investigating that text on your cell phone. Go ahead and click it and see what opens up."

When Brooke did, her "food order" came up with a big green button directing the account holder to "authorize their order" by pressing the button. Brooke pressed the green button, and instantly, a notification came up. "Thank you for your order."

"That's it?" Brooke said.

"That's it. You are now recording." Belinda held up her cell phone and pressed play, and all in the room heard Brooke's question and Belinda's response. Brooke laughed and said, "It seems like I am starring in a Mission Impossible movie."

"Well, we are very high-tech, but you will not be scaling down any 100-story buildings with Tom Cruise," Rhonda interjected.

"Go ahead and press the app again to turn off the recording," Belinda added.

Brooke did, and the same prompts came up to cancel her order.

"Now, talk a bit, and you will hear nothing recorded."

Brooke made some small talk about the weather, and sure enough, when Belinda pulled out her phone, it did not record Brooke's words.

"Ok. I feel comfortable," Brooke said to Rhonda. "Any other tips you can give me?"

"I would wear the transmitter around the rest of the day, so you feel comfortable, and make sure you don't unconsciously look or pull down on your blouse. Plan to forget you have it on and then just have a conversation with the folks at Arch City like you would for anybody accepting a job. Don't ask loaded questions that you think we want answers. Act normal. Act excited about the job. Ask questions on salary, insurance, where your work area is, responsibilities, etc. If there is an opportunity to dig a little deeper, you are a smart woman, and you will know when that presents itself. And remember, activate the transmitter about an hour before your appointment so we can test it again."

Brooke took a deep breath and firmly said to Detective Simon, "I'm ready."

Chapter 59

Vinnie was not ready. In fact, at 8:30 in the morning, he was puking his guts out from too much drinking the afternoon before. After his confrontation with Alex Finnegan, he somehow managed to make it home, where he continued drinking until he passed out, still in the golf clothes he now had vomited all over.

He tried to recall the confrontation with Finnegan the best he could, leaving him more confused. He remembered they talked about the list of donors he now possessed and Finnegan challenging him to do something about it. Most of the conversation was foggy, but the one thing that stood out in his mind was Finnegan telling Vinnie all on the list were terminal and had chosen to die soon, but would it be soon enough to help Frank? What did choosing to die soon mean?"

Trying to sober up the best he could, he took a long shower, then walked down to Shaw's for an espresso and the morning paper. While his head hurt to read, he managed to skim the sports headlines first, then turned to local news. While not looking for any news story, one headline and the two-sentence lead to the story jumped out to him.

Local Businessman Killed in Lake of the Ozarks Boating Accident

Local businessman Steve Darcy, 44, was killed yesterday evening when the boat he was piloting crashed on Lake of the Ozarks.

Usually, a story about a boating accident in the summer at the lake hardly made any news or interested Vinnie. Every summer, at least a dozen people were killed while boating on the lake. Usually, they were drunk, or another drunk boater killed them, but Steve Darcy was one of the people on the donor list, and it was only a few days ago that Vinnie had seen him showing off his new boat to his family.

Vinnie clicked on the whole story and read how the boat, with Mr. Darcy as the sole occupant, had crashed against rocks on the shore at a high rate of speed. There were no details on whether Steve Darcy was drunk or about the cause of the crash., The article did mention that Steve Darcy and his company were currently under an ongoing federal investigation into tax fraud.

Vinnie felt a wave of nausea overcome him, and it was not from the excess booze he had vomited an hour before. He genuinely felt horrible for the family Darcy left behind and was glad none of them were with their husband and father when this terrible accident happened. He thought about how fleeting life was. One minute you are celebrating the purchase of a new boat, life is great, then a few days later, you are dead. The next thought Vinnie had was about another irony in life. Steve Darcy's death could be Frank's salvation. If he was a match, then Frank could be getting his lungs if they were salvageable. What was it that Finnegan said to Vinnie? Something like, "All these people are going to die soon but perhaps not soon enough for Frank." Vinnie's mind raced. Did Finnegan know Darcy was going to die? Did Finnegan cause his death? Did Darcy commit suicide because his company was under investigation?

Regardless of why or how Darcy died, Vinnie, at this moment, did not care. He decided to call Frank, thinking maybe Steve Darcy's death would be Frank's salvation. Sue answered instead. Could that be because Frank was preparing for surgery for the lung transplant Vinnie hoped Darcy would provide? Vinnie was hopeful.

Her voice gave an instant clue that all was not well as she answered the phone.

"Sue, what's wrong?" he asked.

"Hi, Vinnie. You could tell that quickly that I have bad news?"

"Yeah, I could tell. Is something up with Frank?"

"He had an awful night, and his doctor told us to bring him into the hospital last night to prepare for a possible transplant."

"Well, that's good, right?" Vinnie sounded more pleased than he should. "So, they found a donor?"

"No, and to make matters worse, a guy Frank has been rehabbing with just found out that he is getting the lung from a guy who died yesterday afternoon. This morning, we talked to his wife, and she told us her husband was a perfect match with the donor. He is being operated on as we speak. Frank is pretty down. He thought he would be the match for the next donor. Why don't we ever get any good luck?"

Vinnie could tell Sue was holding on tight and holding back from a complete breakdown.

"Sue, what are they saying about Frank? How much time do you think he has to wait before it's too late?"

"I think no more than two weeks. If he does not get a donor by then, I think he will be too far gone, and even if a donor surfaced, Frank might be too weak to survive the operation."

Vinnie was quiet. He was pissed off that Frank did not get the lung that he assumed was donated by the death of Steve Darcy. An angry Vinnie was an unstable Vinnie, and in his gut, he knew he would have to act fast if he was to help Frank at all. He told Sue he would come by to see Frank by 10:00 a.m. and would bring some breakfast treats from the hill. Then he hung up.

Grabbing some pastries and better coffee than they had in the hospital, Vinnie made it to Barnes Hospital a few minutes after ten and quickly made his way up to Frank's room. Once there, he noticed a buzz of activity as Frank was connected to multiple monitors and an oxygen mask to help with his breathing. Several hospital employees were surrounding Frank's bed, and Vinnie sensed he had taken a turn for the worse. Vinnie thought, Is this it? Am I too late?

Soon the employees, Vinnie was unsure if they were nurses, doctors, or aides, walked away from Frank, and as they parted, Vinnie could see Frank's face and his never-ending smile on it. Even if Frank was hours away from death, Vinnie thought Frank would be cheerful.

Seeing Vinnie, Frank waved him over and took off his facemask. "Vinnie, I am glad you finally made it. I want to introduce you to the best nurse in the hospital, Brooke MacIntosh, who runs the transplant floor." Brooke turned to say hello to Vinnie with a megawatt smile and long flowing blonde hair.

"Nice to meet you, Vinnie. Frank has so many friends and relatives. I can't keep them all straight. Are you his brother, brother-in-law?"

"Brother-in-law, Brooke. Nice to meet you, as well. How is this guy doing?"

"He is doing great for a guy who needs some lungs, but I am sure he will be serenading us all here with Italian love songs once he gets them." Frank and Sue both laughed at that, with Sue adding, "I think Brooke's beauty has made Frank delirious as he sings songs in Italian before he falls asleep. But if that is what it takes, sing away, Frank!"

Frank said a small phrase in Italian to Sue and Brooke, who must have picked up small bits of the language dealing with him as she and Sue both laughed.

Brooke began to leave and told Frank they needed to check all his vitals again, and she wanted to see him walk around a bit more. As she left, Vinnie followed her out of the room to ask her a question.

"If you have a minute, Brooke, can I ask you a few questions?"

"Sure, I have a few minutes. What's on your mind?"

"Is Frank going to make it?" Vinnie asked bluntly.

"I would not tell you anything that I have not told Sue and Frank and their family, but Frank is very, very sick, and if he gets lungs, I believe he will make it because he is so strong and has such a great attitude. But he needs lungs and needs them soon."

"Soon like hours, days, weeks?" Vinnie asked.

"We don't like to put a time limit on these things. All I can tell you is Sue and Frank know that most people who need a lung at this stage are brought to the hospital to prepare, and the average stay is about two weeks for either getting lungs or time running out and not getting one. The best thing you can do is pray and keep his spirits up. Is there anything else I can answer for you, Vinnie?"

"No, I guess not. Sometimes, Brooke, we need more than prayer. We don't need divine intervention. We need human intervention."

Brooke looked at Vinnie curiously as what he said seemed so odd to her. Not at all what any other family member would say in this situation. She also thought the statement sounded like something Dr. Finnegan would say about human intervention. She bid Vinnie goodbye and headed down the hallway to check on her other patients.

Vinnie went back into Frank's room as he was getting a comprehensive exam by the medical staff, so Vinnie thought it would be better to leave. After hugging Sue and leaving the room, Vinnie passed a visitor waiting room with a large group of people hugging and crying, but not Vinnie sensed emotions of sorrow but joy. He asked one of the men leaning into the room from the outside corridor what all the commotion was about, and he told Vinnie that his uncle had just received his lung, and they were all celebrating the good news that he was out of surgery and doing well. Vinnie halfheartedly wished the man and his uncle well, and while he had no confirmation that the lung the man received was Steve Darcy's, as it could be anyone's, Vinnie knew that it was one less lung available that could have gone to Frank.

CHAPTER 60

As Detective Simon and Kenny Thorton planned, Kenny arranged another meeting with Antonee the following morning at Bellefontaine Cemetery at 10:30, early enough the cemetery would be quiet but late enough to ensure a guy in Antonee's line of late evening work would show up. Based on Detective Simon's instructions, he knew what to ask Antonee and how to ask without being shot. Detective Simon and a few other plain-clothes cops acted as mournful visitors at several nearby gravesites in case things went south. Due to the sensitive nature of this meeting and to ensure everyone had some familiarity with the grounds of this massive cemetery, Kenny told Antonee to just meet him at the same gravesite they had most recently, William Clark's.

Walking to the tomb, he was surprised to find Antonee and his friends waiting for him. "What's up, man," Antonee greeted Kenny. "Why you need to meet this soon? And what with meeting us at the same dead cracker's hole in the ground we met at the other day? I thought you be like giving us a new history lesson?"

"No history lesson today, Antonee, or at least not an old history lesson about these old white men laying here. Maybe a more recent one. You up for that, Antonee?" Kenny said a little more bravado than he felt right now.

"Ok, ok, I feel you blood. You want to get right down to it, so spit."

"What history are you looking for? But keep in mind, me and my boys, we ain't be giving out free information just because you aks for it."

Kenny said, "Ain't asking for a solid without some cash money on your palms, so how about $1,000 for a little bit. And maybe a few more bills if I like what I hear." Kenny laid ten crisp $100 bills on Antonee's palm.

"Ok, bruh, what you looking for?"

"When you were younger pups, a few years back, I know you guys were running hard with William 'Big Willie' Burroughs and his peeps. Controlling the neighborhood."

"How you be knowing that, Kenny? You not street," Antonee said, glaring a bit more menacingly at Kenny.

Knowing Antonee can go from calm to rage instantly, Kenny calmly said, "I know that because I served prison time for supplying Big Willie the stuff that he and you were selling on the street. I am not sure you knew that Antonee?"

"I heard talk that Big Willie flipped on a doctor who was supplying our dope, but when Big Willie went down, the supply just kept coming, same as before," Antonee said.

"What do you mean same as before, Antonee?" Kenny asked.

Antonee and his boys just laughed, and Antonee, with his grill glimmering in the late morning light, just put out his palm. "Time for another deposit, blood, if you want that juice."

Without hesitation, Kenny laid another $1000 on Antonee's palms.

"Oh, we be doing some good bidness here, my nigga. I say the supply come just like before because nothing changes when you and Big Willie go down. Same schedule, same packs, same dose, same price. It be like you never gone."

"So, Antonee, when Big Willie got out of the joint a few years ago, did everything go back to him? Did he become top-dog on the street again?"

"Hell no. He came back out of the cage, thinking he be back on top, but me and my boys we had something to say about that. He got to earn back his place on the top, or he got to take it from me," Antonee said, then laughing and turning to his two boys, "and we know he not going to be taking anything anymore, is he, my niggas?"

Then moving much closer to Kenny than he was comfortable, Antonee stared at him and said, "You know, Kenny, you starting to ask a few questions that I don't like to hear. You feel me? What you be aiming at, bruh?"

"I'm aiming to get back in the business, Antonee. I know your supply has run dry, right?"

"Well, you know that be true. That why we be selling these insurance policies. Money is clean but not as green as the dope selling."

"Ok, Antonee. Here's what I am going to do for you. I become your new supplier, bringing you about 50% more dope and sell it to you for about 20% less than before."

"Why you give us such a sugar deal, Kenny?" Antonee asked suspiciously.

"Well, you will do something for me to earn this sugar deal. Like Big Willie did to me five years ago, you are going to flip on your former dope supplier to get him behind bars, but not for just dope selling, for accessory to murder."

Defiant, Antonee said, "Hey, bruh, you read me and mine all wrong. We don't snitch. We put the snitch in the ditch if you hear me on that."

"Well, that's fine, too. You turn on this guy, or you put him in a ditch, but either way, you should do it fast. The cops are closing in on him, and he will use you three as leverage to walk, just like he did to me with Big Willie."

"Shit, man, what you talkin' bout? No one got nutin' on us unless we deicides to cap your punk ass right now and have you lay in the dirt next to this cracker," Antonee said, pointing down to William Clark's grave.

"Well, they got something on you, Antonee. You and your crew. They got all three of you leaving a garage downtown after jacking a car and killing a young woman lawyer named Kim DeAngelo. Probably a few days after you killed an old man walking to his car from Busch Stadium - in front of his grandson. Even for you, Antonee, that was cold. And I guess that Big Willie's shooting was done by you as well. But why would you randomly shoot these three people? Or maybe it was not random but ordered by your dope supplier?"

With that comment, all three men pulled their handguns out, aiming directly at Kenny, who held up his hands, not pleading and talking calmer than he imagined. He simply said, "Before you off me, let me ask you something, Antonee. I know the insurance money does not replace the dope money, but my guess is to ensure you are pulling in the large, your former dope supplier is helping you offset that money by giving you another source of green. Like capping some of your brothers in the hood insured by these policies?"

"Well, ain't you some whip-smart cracker? Maybe as smart as the cracker who been taking care of us all these years, but your time above the ground just plain run out," Antonee said, now inching closer to Kenny.

"Well, Antonee, I am smart enough to know not to have this conversation with you alone. You might want to know there are cameras all over this cemetery, probably four pointing at you right now, and you might want to look to your right and left. Those mourners over there, putting flowers on those graves, seem to be packing heat. You kill me now, Antonee, you and yours will 100% get executed in prison, but you help me now, you won't walk away clean, but you won't die in the joint, either. Who knows? With packed jails, you may get out in 15 years, still young enough to have time for plenty more crimes and jail in your life."

Detective Simon and four undercover cops, guns drawn, rushed to Kenny, Antonee, and his boys. Kenny knew this could turn bad as their street instincts were never to surrender but blast their way out. But Antonee and his crew just dropped their guns, and Antonee said to Kenny, "I ain't be taking the needle for no cracker, Kenny. I might tell the pigs all about the dude who give us the word to move on, that lawyer, the old man, and the boys. I may be in a talking mood, but me and my boys gotta have a deal, Kenny."

Detective Simon and her team had taken control of Antonee and his crew and were headed down to the precinct to see what kind of deal they could make to get them to flip on Alex Finnegan.

CHAPTER 61

Brooke got dressed, checked the wire, and by 3:00 was leaving her apartment for the meeting with Dr. Calabrese at 3:30. Walking into The Center, she knew this visit would turn out differently than her last visit when she was taking a tour. But she was ready for anything Dr. Calabrese would say to her. A welcome sign greeted her, and when she checked in, she was greeted warmly by the receptionist, who welcomed her to the Arch City team. She then gave Brooke directions to Dr. Calabrese's office and told her to head up as Dr. Calabrese was expecting her.

Brooke took the elevator to Dr. Calabrese's office. Her office was bright and pleasant, accented with modern décor and beautiful flowers bathed in sunlight from the floor-to-ceiling windows overlooking Forest Park.

Dr. Calabrese got up from behind her desk and warmly welcomed Brooke with a handshake and a slight hug. All past meetings with Dr. Calabrese were a bit more formal, so this personal touch caught Brooke slightly off guard.

"Brooke, it seems it has been a long time since we first met here, but I am so glad you have decided to accept our offer and will be joining the Arch City Transplant team."

Brooke gave Ellen a pleasant smile and said, "Ellen, it is nice to be here. I am very excited by the opportunity and look forward to joining you and Dr. Finnegan."

"Great, Brooke. Please sit down. We will need an hour of your time to begin all the paperwork and get you ready for your start date, and I am sure you have lots of questions for us. However, before we start, did you bring the employment contract we provided you?"

Brooke pulled out the contract and handed it to Ellen, who glanced at it and then placed it on her desk. Turning back to Brooke, she asked, "Before I begin, do you have any questions?"

Brooke knew not to jump in right away with some of the questions Detective Simon wanted her to broach about TTWC, so she stayed on script and talked only about the impending job, asking about salary, 401K, insurance, hours, etc. She did ask that she be able to give the hospital at least three weeks' notice saying her replacement would need training. Dr. Calabrese was agreeable to all of Brooke's requests. Then Brooke decided to ask a few more questions about her specific duties, and in her mind, she had a pathway of questions to ask Dr. Calabrese that would hopefully give Detective Simon what she was seeking. Brooke looked down at her blouse, wondering if the wire was visible. Dr. Calabrese did not seem to notice, so Brooke relaxed and proceeded.

"Ellen, I know my title is Director of Transplant Synergy, and at a 10,000-foot level, I understand what that entails, but can you get more into the specifics about what you expect of me in the position?"

"Sure, Brooke. I would describe your job in two ways. One way being internal and the other external. Whenever possible, our goal is to bring donors and recipients together before a transplant occurs. You had seen this interaction in the family room when you came on your tour."

Brooke nodded in affirmation.

"While that is a big piece of your job, ensuring the smooth interaction between donors and recipients, it is only a small piece and the one I would call an internal job requirement. But it is not the most important part of your job. That would be the external aspects, the community outreach, so to speak. As you know, everything in the transplant process works well when you have ample donors to meet the demands of the recipients, but society doesn't have ample donors. Our mission, your job, if you will, at The Center, is to raise the level of donors in general and specifically ones that will use The Center when the time of donation is near."

Brooke, although knowing this is what Alex had covered with her at dinner a few nights back, let Ellen continue and asked, "How do I do that? Do you have plans in place?"

"Yes and no," Ellen responded. "Because what we are trying to do is so groundbreaking, so outside the norm, that while we are improving traditional methods of increasing donors, we need to try new methods."

"Such as?" Brooke said, trying to lead Ellen to answer the question she was about to ask.

"Such as community outreach in churches, assisted living facilities, nursing homes, and even AA-type meetings, all places that influence a person's decision to become a donor. You would go to the places and hopefully, speak to groups or individuals about the shortage of donors and then talk about the mission of The Center. It's a unique position, Brooke. We think your background in the medical side of transplants and your persuasive personality could be a real difference-maker for us."

Brooke knew she had to ask her questions soon as the time was becoming short, and she had run out of general subjects to talk to Ellen about. So, it was time to take a chance and see if she could trip up Dr. Calabrese.

"That is very interesting, Ellen. So, what involvement would I have with TTWC, the insurance company connected to The Center through organ donations?"

"Brooke, I told you at lunch a few weeks back that those women who mentioned The Center could have been talking about anything. Not necessarily associated with us."

Brooke nodded at Ellen and said, "Actually, Ellen, The Center has a direct connection to TTWC."

"How so, Brooke?" Ellen cautiously asked, knowing she was getting into an area she was unprepared to discuss with Brooke.

"I was visiting a friend of mine who is an ER doc, and while she was tending to a gunshot victim, I sat with the victim's mother. While we were waiting for the police to interview her about the shooting, she showed me an insurance policy from TTWC and told me she would be paid $50,000 if she could get her son's body to The Center to take out his parts, which I assume meant to be his organs."

Ellen, her tone a bit more exasperated, said, "Brooke, as I told you before, The Center can mean anything. What proof do you have it is our Center?"

Brooke picked up her phone, scrolled to her photos, and showed Ellen the policy, which pointed out the organs must be donated to The Arch Transplant Center.

Ellen said nothing. Brooke was unsure if Ellen was totally surprised by the connection or knew about it all along and was planning her next lie.

Finally, breaking the silence and the instructions Detective Simon specifically warned her about, Brooke said, "Dr. Calabrese, in every meeting I have had with you and Dr. Finnegan, I have been both impressed and afraid of your approaches. I understand you must push the envelope to have breakthroughs in medicine, especially transplants, so I was very interested in your job offer. I saw you both as visionaries. But now I see you as something else."

Interrupting, Ellen said, "Brooke, we are visionaries, and everything we are doing, while edgy and controversial, are in our minds legally defensible, and I assure you if they were not, I would not be involved with The Center."

"Interesting, Doctor. So, murder is now controversial and edgy? Why? Because it is for the greater good? For the big picture?"

Ellen's voice uncharacteristically rose in anger. "We have told you that we believe our approach to using physician-assisted suicide to find more donors is legally defensible because it is for the greater good. And, it is the choice we are allowing terminal people to make. What you and others may claim to be murder is rather, in our opinion, acts of mercy to both allow those to die with dignity while also giving them a choice to use their organs as they wish and to whom they wish."

"That is not what I am talking about. However, you are straddling the moral fence with that position. I am talking about killing the people insured on TTWC policies."

With anger subsiding and replaced with an exaggerated laugh, Ellen said, "Brooke, you can't be serious. There is no way we would be involved in something like that. We are doctors, not murderers."

Looking at Ellen directly and calmly, Brooke reached for her employment application, took it off Ellen's desk, and said, "You won't need this. I've decided to pass on your generous offer." Then as she was getting up to leave, Brooke gave Ellen Detective Simon's card and said, "But you may need this because if you are unaware of TTWC's true purpose, you may want to clear your name."

Five miles away at her office, Detective Simon turned off the recording. Rhonda thought Brooke MacIntosh was a woman to be taken very seriously and that she was going places in her life. While the street thugs gave her enough evidence to arrest Alex Finnegan for the murders of Thomson, DeAngelo, and Burroughs, Rhonda needed more decisive confirmation because Finnegan had powerful connections in the city. Because of Brooke's aggressive and risky approach, Rhonda felt she was close to pinning Finnegan and perhaps Calabrese to the killings of those poor souls insured by TTWC. Murders caused by the greed and God complex of both Doctors, whose credo was "Do No Harm.".

CHAPTER 62

Sitting at home after visiting Frank, Vinnie was already hitting the bourbon hard despite it being only 1:00 p.m. He looked down at his phone and saw a text from a number that seemed somewhat familiar, and after reading the text, chills went up his spine.

"Too bad Steve Darcy died and was not a perfect match for Frank. One down, three to go. Act fast, Vinnie. Frank's days are numbered and so are yours!"

The text came from the same number initially contacting him to meet at the Grand Basin to receive the donor list. He now knew that the list came from Finnegan, through an intermediary, and now this text. Finnegan was messing with Vinnie's mind, but what was his end game? It could not be to help Frank. Was it to goad Vinnie into doing something with one of these donors? But if so, what would Finnegan get out of it?

He repeatedly returned to Finnegan's comment: "They are going to die anyways but may not be in time to save your brother-in-law."

Vinnie thought it best to try and learn why everyone on the list would die soon. This would be delicate, but he had bullshitted his way into Marvin Applebaum and Jonas Stecker's world, so he thought meeting Raul Montez now made sense.

Vinnie headed down to the Wash U campus again, parking offsite so security cameras would less likely see his truck and walked again to the

School of Architecture, where he had sat in Montez's lecture. He went back to the lecture hall and popped his head in, hoping to see if Dr. Montez was teaching, but giving a lecture was an older female professor. Walking out of the hall, he asked a student where Dr. Montez's office was, and the student cheerfully directed him to the professor's office on the first floor of the building. Vinnie was thinking about a plausible story for him to get into Dr. Montez's office to either look around or begin asking him questions. As he walked by the office door, he noticed the lights off, indicating Montez was not in the office. Wandering through the hallway, Vinnie came to a reception area where a young woman diligently worked the keyboard on her laptop.

"Excuse me, Miss. I am wondering if you can tell me if Professor Montez is around?"

"I don't believe he is but let me check his schedule," she said as she opened what seemed to be several more screens on her laptop. Scrolling down on the page, she must have come to Professor Montez's full schedule because she said, "No, I am sorry, sir. Dr. Montez is out of the office for the next month."

"Ok," Vinnie said. "That seems odd, considering classes are in session. Do you know where he is or how I may be able to reach him?"

Looking up at him, she said, "No, sir. I am sorry. I have no other information I can give you."

Vinnie thought a minute. He was about to leave, but another nearby student walked up to Vinnie and said, "Sir, I overheard you asking about Dr. Montez, and I am not sure if what you need is important, but he is in Asia and for the most part unreachable."

"Asia. Why would he be in Asia?" Vinnie asked.

Now speaking very quietly so no one would overhear them, the student said, "Dr. Montez is on a bucket-list trip, touring some of the great urban architecture in Asia. It was always his dream he did that before he passed."

"Is he sick?" Vinnie asked, stating the obvious but trying to see if any more valuable information would be forthcoming. The student just replied, "We all hope we get to see him again, but I am not so sure that we will."

Vinnie just thought. Darcy is dead. Montez is unreachable, and when or if he got back to the states, would it be too late for Vinnie?

Two donor options are left. Frank's odds were getting worse.

CHAPTER 63

Rhonda knew she had Kenny Thorton as leverage over Finnegan, but she needed more. While Antonee and his boys had flipped on Alex, she knew Alex still had powerful men in his camp. They had so much to lose they would do anything legal or illegal to manipulate the legal system to ensure the three gang members were the ones convicted, and Alex Finnegan walked away free. Based on Brooke's conversation with Dr. Ellen Calabrese, Simon knew Dr. Calabrese was the critical person to ensnare Finnegan, so even his backers could not or would not want to free him. Of course, Rhonda was still unsure whether Calabrese was in lock step with Finnegan on this, but an accomplice to murder, for someone like Dr. Calabrese, seemed to be quite the reach. However, Rhonda knew that money and power made people do crazy things.

Rhonda did not want Dr. Calabrese to be defensive or embarrassed that a Detective showed up at her place of work, her domain, to question her. So, Rhonda decided to call Dr. Calabrese's office instead and asked to speak with her. After being screened about the nature of the call, Rhonda, without using her name and knowing HIPPA regulations would stop anyone from prying, just said the call was a private health matter. Seconds later, Rhonda connected to Dr. Calabrese, who answered in a pleasant and professional voice,

"Hello, this is Dr. Calabrese. How can I help you?"

"Hello, Doctor. I am Detective Rhonda Simon from the St. Louis PD. Perhaps you were expecting my call?"

"Yes, unfortunately, I was Detective, but before I say anything more, tell me why I should not hang up and get our lawyers involved in this."

"You have the right to do that, Doctor, but I am not placing you under arrest or anything like that. I am just calling to ask you some questions you may want to listen to before you call your lawyers who might give you some bad advice, depending on whether they are in your camp or Dr. Finnegan's."

Ellen took note of that comment. She knew that The Center's lawyers were all long-time cronies of Alex's, and if push came to shove, they would push her under the bus to protect Alex.

"I am comfortable talking to you alone, Detective, but let's do it away from my office, in about an hour at the Starbucks right around the corner in Maryland Plaza. Do you know the one?"

"Yes, I do. I will see you in a bit." Rhonda said as she hung up the phone, planning to get to Starbucks a few minutes early to look around a bit to make sure she could find a quiet place to talk.

Arriving at the Starbucks, which had its usual flow of customers, most drinking coffee and transfixed on a laptop or cell phone, Rhonda decided the best place would be a table outside, as the afternoon sun had begun to weaken. A cool breeze made a shady spot somewhat bearable for a summer day. Although tolerable, it was still hot. So, Rhonda opted for iced tea instead of hot coffee and, knowing Dr. Calabrese was probably walking here from The Center, ordered her one as well, grabbing an extra cup of ice and some sweetener.

Fifty minutes had passed since she hung up with Dr. Calabrese. Knowing how badly doctors kept schedules, she assumed she would be waiting for a while. But looking up, she saw an elegant and professionally dressed woman heading her way that she believed was Dr. Calabrese. Dr. Calabrese pegged Rhonda as the Detective she was meeting and headed straight towards her with her hand extended.

"Detective Simon, I presume. Hi, I am Dr. Calabrese."

"Pleasure to meet you, Doctor," Rhonda said, noting Ellen did not ask Rhonda to be less formal with titles. "I hope you don't mind, but I thought this outside table would be a quiet place to talk, and I think tolerable with the breeze and shade. I also got you an iced tea instead of coffee, handing her the cold plastic glass."

"Perfect, thank you. I can't drink coffee on these hot days and never got into iced coffee. So, iced tea is great, and sitting outside is fine. I know we are supposedly past the worst of Covid, and that's great, but whenever I can, I still like to sit outside versus inside," Ellen said pleasantly.

Rhonda noticed Ellen's ease and comfort with her, similar to her first meeting with Kenny Thorton. In her experience, innocent people with nothing to hide are more at ease than guilty ones, except sociopaths, and Dr. Calabrese did not seem to be a sociopath.

"Doctor, I will get right to the point because I know you are busy," Rhonda waded in.

"Yes, thank you for that, Detective. I have a dinner meeting with the board and Alex in about 90 minutes, so I need to get home and change for that. But I live close and can spend about 30 minutes with you.

Rhonda debated how hard and fast to get into this with Ellen, but since her next meeting was with Alex and the board, she decided to go in hard and fast and use shock to motivate Ellen to be forthcoming.

"Are you aware of Dr. Finnegan's friendship with a man named Kenny Thorton?"

"Yes, they go way back. They were medical school roommates, and I think they may have been in business together five or six years ago at some clinic."

"Are you aware of them being business associates, in fact, partners, now?"

"No, I am unaware of any business partnership Alex would have with Kenny. I would be surprised because Alex knows Kenny is a loose cannon and trouble, as far as I am concerned. I know Alex gives Kenny some odd jobs now and then to help him out after he lost his medical license, but I don't think anything more substantive than that."

While it might have been the late afternoon heat versus nervousness, Rhonda did notice tiny beads of perspiration form on Ellen's face. Rhonda wondered how much Ellen knew about Alex and Kenny's arrangement.

"Doctor, how familiar are you with why Kenny Thorton lost his license and the business Dr. Finnegan, and he once had?"

"I know Kenny Thorton was and is, who knows, a drug addict, and he got caught selling prescription opioids on the street. That's why he lost his license. I don't know much about their business because I did not know them then." Looking at her watch, Ellen added, "Detective, it seems you are more interested in Kenny Thorton, so why don't you talk to him instead of me."

"Oh, I have. Kenny is doing quite well for himself. I am surprised you did not know this, but Kenny is President of TTWC Insurance company, the same company that has a contract with The Center to supply organs of those who pass and insured by TTWC."

Ellen looked surprised, and while outwardly her emotions remained in check, internally, she was starting to boil as she knew anything involved with Kenny Thorton was trouble. Coolly she said, "That news surprises me, Detective, although there are facets of the business under Alex's domain, not mine. I oversee medical operations."

Ellen was very much in control, so to not lose her, Rhonda pushed again.

"Doctor, let me tell you something else you may not know about Dr. Finnegan and Kenny Thorton's history. Do you know that Kenny Thorton, while found guilty of opioid selling, ended up in prison because his great buddy Alex Finnegan turned on him to cover his own hide?"

"Hearsay and ancient history as far as I'm concerned, Detective."

"Ok, let me modernize this for you. Over the last several months, three people involved in the opioid case against Kenny Thorton turned up dead. The opioid distributor, who fingered Kenny for a reduced sentence, the prosecuting attorney, and a private investigator."

"It would seem to me that Kenny Thorton is on a little revenge killing tour, wouldn't it, Detective?" Ellen asked a little too smugly for Rhonda's taste. Rhonda, at this point, did not like Dr. Calabrese and was hoping she was involved because she would love to wipe the smugness off her face.

"Doctor, the average lay person would jump to that conclusion, but murder is not always what it seems. I now have three killers in jail who identified Alex Finnegan as the person who instructed them to do the killings. The people they murdered knew of Finnegan's involvement in the Life Health Center opioid trafficking, and they knew Finnegan was no innocent bystander. Information my guess that would be devastating, at this point, in Finnegan's life and business success."

"That's preposterous, Detective!" Ellen said loud enough that nearby patrons turned in her direction. Then more quietly, she said, "I can say with 100% conviction that Kenny would be more prone to do something like this than Alex. Maybe these killers you have in custody are working with Kenny, covering his tracks. My God, Detective! Do you know what type of man you are accusing?"

Rhonda firmly replied, "I know the exact type of man Alex Finnegan is. A man who believes laws do not apply if they get in the way of his goals. No different than any street punk in my experience. But I wondered if they were covering for Kenny. That would make more sense, but they confessed to one more crime which in my mind unequivocally ties back to Dr. Finnegan and maybe you."

Sensing Dr. Calabrese was about to bolt or lawyer up, Rhonda played her last card, hoping it would win this poker game.

"Dr. Calabrese, I know this is all shocking, and you probably think it is time to shut up and get your lawyers involved, but that is what a guilty person would do. While I am not convinced yet of your implication in this, please listen to what I have on Finnegan. If you are not involved, you can come out of this clean and prosperous."

"Ok, Detective. You have five minutes before I am out of here," Ellen said firmly.

"The killers who confessed to the killings of those involved with the Life Health Center case are some of the people selling the TTWC life insurance policies, but they also confessed to killing some of the insured policy owners, again at the direction of Alex Finnegan."

Ellen sat in silence, stunned, knowing that Brooke had also brought this accusation up.

Rhonda continued, "From what I understand from Kenny Thorton, Finnegan has so much riding on making The Center a success that he is taking huge chances to create more donors and donors nobody would miss. Poor black men killed in the inner city."

Ellen just sat back and thought of all the late-night conversations she had with Alex about The Center, its goals, and the obstacles to reaching those goals. She knew Alex was pushing moral boundaries with the 'My Body, My Choice' cultural reckoning, but she never thought he would do something as immoral as killing innocent people for their organs. But was anything out of bounds for Alex? He always talked about the greed and depravity of humanity and that anyone would do anything for love or money, but would Alex be a killer for money? She knew he loved power more than anything and felt he could control any situation. The more she thought about Alex's thirst for power, the more she convinced herself that perhaps Alex could be involved in all of this.

Snapping out of her silent and darkening thoughts, Ellen heard Detective Simon ask, "Dr. Calabrese, you and Dr. Finnegan, the board, and the investors are sitting on a goldmine if what I read about The Center comes true. You own many shares and will become wealthy if The Center succeeds. Correct?"

"Detective, based on news about The Center, our investor commitment, and projected capitalization rate when and if we go public, you know what the future could have in store for us. So, yes. If The Center succeeds, I will become very rich," Ellen answered factually but not boastfully.

Rhonda continued, "And if Alex Finnegan were to get convicted of a crime, one of two things could happen. One, the investors pull out, and The Center folds like a cheap tent or two; if you are clean, you take the helm, right the ship, and The Center and all the future riches are protected, assuming you are also not involved with TTWC and the murders of those insured."

"I am not involved in anything," Ellen said firmly. "The picture you just painted outlines two scenarios, one bad for Alex, myself, and The Center and one bad for Alex but has me coming out on top. The latter scenario flatters me and, perhaps in your mind, motivates me to help you find out if Alex is guilty. Detective, what you don't know about me, is I could care less if my stock is worthless if Alex is guilty of a crime. I would be the first to call you if I found out Alex was involved in these murders. My work and reputation are more important to me than any multimillion-dollar payout The Center might provide down the road."

"Well, maybe a billion-dollar payout, but I respect your integrity and honesty, Dr. Calabrese. However, if you are innocent, you need to help us with Alex Finnegan, which will be the only way to clear your name. Let me ask you a question. Do you trust him? Do you think if his ass were on the line, he would turn on you, as he did with Kenny, his best friend, five years ago to protect himself?"

Dr. Calabrese thought for a minute, then answered Rhonda, "What I know about Alex is he is brilliant, driven, and an ego manic, like most men in his position. I also know that any man like Alex believes they are invincible, and pushing the envelope legally and ethically motivates him, but that is a long way from being a murderer."

"Doctor, with all due respect, I have put hundreds of men in jail who have the same attributes and did, in fact, murder someone they felt was threatening their lifestyle, whether modest or grand. Everyone is capable of murder, Dr. Calabrese, especially Alex Finnegan, who has so much to lose. He is capable of anything, and he will destroy the lives of the innocent, including yours and Kenny's, once more, to get what he wants. When you look deep into Alex Finnegan's eyes, what do you see, Dr. Calabrese? Do you see innocence, compassion, caring for those around him?"

Ellen thought for a minute, then said, "Excuse me for a second, Detective," and picked up her cell phone and started texting. When she finished texting, she turned to Rhonda, "I told Alex I would be late for cocktails, so he should start without me. You have me for thirty more minutes to convince me I should trust you and not Alex."

CHAPTER 64

The next day, after contemplating the news about Raul Montez, Vinnie began to sense some urgency as fate, or as Frank's continued bad luck would have it, two potential donors were no longer viable options for Frank. Steve Darcy had died, and Vinnie assumed his family had donated his organs. Raul Montez was out of the country for a month, and by the time he got back, if he got back, Frank might be dead.

Vinnie pulled up the online music schedule for local bars and saw that Brothers Roosevelt, the band in which Jonas Stecker played sax, was playing at Hammerstone's tonight. He got there at the tail end of the set, hoping that Brittany, the bartender, would not be there. While flattered with her interest, he did not need her as a complication tonight.

Vinnie tried to enjoy himself and the music as the band played an excellent compilation of blues and jazz, some classic tunes, and some newer original material. Jonas Stecker was a passable sax player, but just like during the day, his facial expression indicated angst, not depicting the joy of playing and getting lost in a jam.

Vinnie had never played a musical instrument, but he always admired musicians and thought to himself that being a working musician would be the best job in the world. But Jonas Stecker did not seem to enjoy his night or day job. In Vinnie's mind, Jonas Stecker was one of those guys who did not appreciate all the talents God had given him and instead wasted his life.

The last set finished at midnight, an hour of the night that Vinnie usually would be fast asleep. Vinnie was not sure he could stay awake much longer, so he hoped that Stecker would not hang around till the bar closing time at 1:00. Fortunately, Vinnie could see Stecker's relationship with the band was as aloof as it was with his daytime coworkers. He could tell by the packing of instruments and body language that while the band may stick around for a few late-night beers, Stecker was not interested in any comradery. As Stecker said his goodbyes, Vinnie quickly downed his beer, threw a $20 on the bar, and headed out to his car to watch for Stecker's exit. After a few minutes, Stecker left the bar and went to his bicycle chained to a pole. He unlocked the chain, hopped on his bike, and headed south past Soulard Market to his apartment, which Vinnie knew was less than a mile away on Sidney Street. Vinnie followed but kept his distance because at this time of night, with the street empty, following too close would alarm Stecker.

Vinnie was twitchy, nervous about what to do with Jonas Stecker but believing, in his mind, that Stecker seemed to be a real asshole. Vinnie rationalized that Jonas Stecker had done all he would ever do in this life, and maybe, just maybe, his death would be the only contribution Stecker would ever make to society. And certainly, Vinnie rationalized, Frank's life was worth more than Jonas Stecker's life. As Vinnie followed Stecker, he remembered the guy in the park a month or so ago who died from a hit and run while riding his bike and assumed that guy's organs were donated. As a lone bike rider riding on the dark streets of Soulard, Stecker was almost asking to be hit by a car. The more Stecker rode, the more Vinnie convinced himself Stecker dying could be the solution for Frank.

Stecker continued south on 9th street towards the Anheuser-Busch brewery, and Vinnie assumed he would be taking a right on Sidney Street unless he decided to stop at any of the bars still open. He could not take the chance of Jonas choosing to be social and did not want to get too close to Stecker's apartment, where nosy neighbors might still be awake. Vinnie knew he had to make his move before Stecker turned off 9th street, where the area bordered the ball fields of the Gene Slay Boys and Girls Club of

St. Louis and had the most open space between business and residential dwellings. "Now or never," Vinnie kept saying. "Now or never."

Vinnie stepped on the gas and briefly closed his eyes, saying under his breath, "This is for you, Frank. This is for you." After hitting him with his truck, Vinnie stopped the car and looked back to see what damage he had done. Seeing his bike on the pavement and Stecker's body flat on the sidewalk a few feet away, he knew he had hit him hard enough to cause what he hoped was an injury that would put him close to death. Because Vinnie needed Stecker's body found quickly, he called 911 immediately to report that he had seen a man injured on the sidewalk. He hung up immediately before the 911 dispatcher could ask him his name.

CHAPTER 65

A day had gone by, and still no news of the hit and run of Jonas Stecker. So, Vinnie decided to try and find out for himself what may have happened. He decided to go back to Hammerstone's and see if the bartender Brittany or any other employees might have heard anything about Stecker.

He needed to be careful and avoid asking directly about him, but he felt he had to get a sense if any news about Stecker had reached the restaurant. Walking in and taking a seat at the bar, he was glad to see that Brittany was on shift again. The bar was more crowded in the early evening than it had been at lunch, but Brittany noticed him and gave him a nod that she would be by to get him a drink shortly. Vinnie took a seat at the far end of the bar.

After a few minutes, Brittany came by to take his order. "What will the jazz man have this evening?"

"How about a black and tan to start?" Vinnie replied.

Pouring the ale and stout combo expertly, Brittany placed it in front of Vinnie and, as she did, asked, "So, did you make it here last night to catch the music? I didn't see you."

Vinnie did not know whether to lie and say he did not make it. He thought he would gain nothing by lying and would probably have to explain himself if somehow someone working now had seen him last night.

"I did make it by here but was later than planned. I did catch the last set of the band. They were pretty good, and your bartender friend wasn't too bad of a sax player."

The comment got an instant reaction from Brittany as she put her head down for a moment, then leaned into Vinnie, telling him quietly, "Probably not my place to tell a stranger this, but last night Jonas got hit by a car on his bike going home."

Vinnie wanted to express concern but not too much interest as he did not know Stecker, and it would be odd for him to offer anything more than general thoughts. "Oh man, that sucks. Any word on how he's doing?"

Brittany, casually wiping down an already clean bar in front of Vinnie, shook her head and said, "I hear he's on life support at Barnes."

In a very sympathetic tone, Vinnie said, "I am sorry to hear that. I know you said he could be kind of an ass, but that doesn't deserve to happen to anyone."

"Thanks, jazz man. Hey, if you need anything else, give me a nod. Kind of busy, so please be patient." Brittany shifted down the bar and started taking orders from other patrons as he sat looking at his beer glass half-filled.

He thought he had expressed the right amount of concern to Brittany about Stecker, but deep inside, he was elated. Draining his beer, he caught Brittany's eye and threw a $20 down for a $10 tab. Vinnie headed home, hoping to sleep better, hoping that Frank would soon receive an organ but in the back of his mind, he began to think that perhaps he had made a huge mistake.

CHAPTER 66

T he morning after Ellen's conversation with Detective Simon and subsequent dinner with Alex and the investors, Ellen's eyes began to open a bit more about the real Alex Finnegan. Detective Simon painted a disturbing image of Alex in her mind. While she was always uncomfortable with Alex's willingness to push the envelope in business, she always eventually agreed with him. His potential involvement in a murder scared the hell out of Ellen, both impacting the future of The Center as well as potentially Ellen's life. She was sure that Alex would implicate anyone, including her, if it would save his ass.

As she watched Alex hold court last night, cigar in one hand, brandy in another, telling boastful stories to his board and investors on the success he and The Center would have, she began to see Alex in a new light. Not as a medical and business genius, but as a cunning diabolical criminal who would screw over, even perhaps murder, anyone who would get in his way. His god-complex convinced Alex he was untouchable, irreplaceable. Alex's investors lapped up everything Alex said, and Ellen was sure if he asked them for another five million that night, they would have gladly given it to him. Ellen wondered if Alex was also taking the investors for a ride. It would be dangerous for Alex to do so as these men were some of the wealthiest and most powerful men in St. Louis and the country.

After Detective Simon laid out what she had on Alex, and after Ellen passionately and hopefully convincingly pleaded her innocence, they accepted a mutual trust. They began developing a plan allowing Ellen to confront Alex Finnegan directly. For all the years she had known him, she had put up with his arrogance and ego because beneath it all, she felt he, and the vision of The Center, would save thousands of lives as it would improve the archaic process of organ donations. And while Alex sometimes belittled Ellen and had traditional chauvinistic attitudes toward her and many women, she also knew that Alex's success would mean a financial windfall for her, so she put up with his shit.

Ellen strode into his office where Alex sat alone with his Air Pods in his ears, listening to classical music, Ellen presumed, probably Vivaldi, Alex's preferred choice. As he waved to her to sit down, he listened for a few more seconds before taking the headphones off. Ellen said,

"Vivaldi, Summer concerto?"

"The Winter concerto to take my mind off this never-ending heatwave. What brings you by, Ellen?"

Ellen had no plans to ease into the conversation with Alex. She wanted to hit him hard with accusations as she did not want his mind to begin racing ahead to spin a tale to satisfy Ellen.

"Tell me about your past business with Life Health Center and Kenny Thorton."

"That was years ago, Ellen, and it's a subject in which I am no longer interested. Next question."

"No, let's stay on this one. Do the names Kim DeAngelo, Bill Thomson, and William Burroughs ring a bell for you?"

"No, never heard of them. Ellen, I am swamped, so if you don't have anything else..."

The first lie, Ellen thought.

"You know all three were murdered in the last month, and all three were connected to the case against Life Health Center and Kenny's conviction of opioid dealing?"

This news got Alex's attention as he said, "Murdered. Oh, no. What did that idiot Kenny do now?"

Second lie.

"I am not sure Kenny did anything. Perhaps you are more involved with these murders than Kenny."

"Be very careful, Ellen. You are accusing your boss of some very serious and frankly wild accusations, and my question is, why do you give a rat's ass about Kenny? You hate him."

"Yeah, I am not Kenny's biggest fan. I think he is a loser, but I am asking because I want to know what you did to save your ass and screw Kenny five years ago during that case."

"You know, Ellen, you seem to be asking questions about a subject you would know nothing about. It's almost as if someone has something on you, and you are here to entrap me. Are you here to entrap me, Ellen? Are you here to trick me into telling some wild tale of my involvement with Kenny? Maybe you should unbutton your blouse so I can ensure you are not wearing a wire," laughed Alex.

"Fuck you, Alex. You pig," Ellen seethed.

Unrattled and with a growing smirk on his face, Alex replied, "Well, maybe we will get that blouse off you some time. But why the interest in Kenny and our business together years ago?"

"My interest is to understand why, based on Kenny's past, you would get into bed with him again, forming TTWC, the insurance company that brings those who die to our Center to harvest their organs?"

"Fine, I did that, but I did not tell you because you wanted plausible deniability from certain aspects of our business, remember, Ellen? I did it to help Kenny because he is a friend, maybe my only real friend, and he would do anything for me. Giving him TTWC was effective because the way I set it up ensures Kenny prospers, but also any questionable actions taken by TTWC don't stick to The Center or me."

For a man who ten minutes ago was condescending and arrogant, he now was trying to convince Ellen how humane he was, how much he wanted to help his friend. Ellen thought this side of Alex was more sickening than his arrogance.

"Well, Alex, maybe helping Kenny was an honorable decision, but you made a bad decision when you used his thug TTWC agents to murder the last three people who knew what you did to Kenny so many years ago at Life Health Center."

"You have it all wrong. It is more likely Kenny is the one who ordered the killings of all those people. All of them helped get him convicted. It's his revenge. Kenny even told me the police questioned him after seeing his car near all the murder scenes. That makes more sense. Can't you see that?"

"On the surface, that certainly makes more sense, but those three guys sang quite loudly to the police how your hand was the hand paying for the murders of DeAngelo, Thomson, and Burroughs."

Still, without any anger or fear, Alex said with his usual arrogance, "Now remember who you are talking to. It sounds like you have been spending too much time streaming Netflix. Either that or you have a wild imagination."

"Alex, on the path you are going, you will have plenty of time to let your imagination run wild as you will be whiling away the hours in a prison cell. But unfortunately, I don't think they get Netflix in prison."

"Ellen, Ellen, Ellen. I told you, people like me don't go to prison for our crimes if I committed a crime, which I didn't. We write books, do speaking tours, and get appointed to boards. Not prison, not me."

"You are a smug, condescending asshole," Ellen grumbled at Alex.

"I have had enough of these questions and you, you ungrateful bitch. I am still your boss or was, but you have outlived your usefulness. You are fired," Alex said with his voice now rising in anger.

Showing no concern, Ellen pushed harder into Alex. "Well, you can fire me now, but I will get my job back. No, I'll get a new position, your position, because I set up a meeting with the board and investors who will soon listen to a fascinating story about you." She wanted Alex to know she was going all-in on the hand she was playing.

"The board is in my pocket. They won't believe anything you say," Alex seethed.

"Well, at the meeting, I will have some backup. People you know and people you don't, who will not have just theories, but they will also have evidence to prove everything we have just talked about.

Alex snapped back, "Who? Who is your backup, and what bullshit evidence would they have?"

"You know Kenny Thorton, of course. He has some interesting stories and a few documents that might make you squirm a bit. It seems he is ready to turn on you. The other person is Detective Rhonda Simon. You don't know her, but you will be meeting her soon as she has sworn testimony by the men you hired to commit not only the three murders of those connected to your involvement in the Life Health Clinic but also the murders of young men who TTWC insured."

Still playing it cool, Alex said, "So, you have some gang bangers and a convicted drug dealer as your witnesses. Not a very strong hand, Ellen. I think my reputation and connections will get whatever case the cops may have against me thrown out at once. We will lock the gang bangers up, and everyone is happy."

"You mean you will make a deal like you did to throw Kenny under the bus five years ago at Life Health Clinic? That was easy to pull off because nobody cared if Kenny and Life Health Clinic went down, but your connections, many of the men investing heavily in The Center, have a little more at stake. Financially, politically, personally, if they don't get in front of this thing. None of them will have your back, Alex. You are a big liability, and while you did not pull any triggers, you are still a murderer."

Now there was a change in tone from Alex as he took a different tack.

He said, "Ellen, think about this and what it could mean to you. I can easily pin the murders of DeAngelo, Thomson, and Burroughs on Kenny. He is the logical suspect with a prime motive. As far as the murders of those insured by TTWC, all that did was make The Center more successful, more quickly, and our investors even richer. If I had some inner-city kids killed, so what? They would probably die anyway, and I just sped up the inevitable and cleaned up the streets. When they became organ donors, we made $250,000 on each organ we transplanted, which equaled $2,000,000 per donor. I think our investors and our board would like that return on their investment."

"That is despicable, Alex. You are a doctor, and your first promise as a doctor is to do no harm."

"True, Ellen, but it's not me doing harm. It is our society that has made certain lives meaningless and disposable. I am just creating efficiency in the process to make money."

"So, preying on the underserved, the poor, minorities are ok because their lives are meaningless?" Ellen asked with frustration and anger in her voice.

"Not just the people at the bottom of the barrel. We are also creating efficiency for those who have lived a good life and have contributed to society. They have already contributed in life, but they can make more contributions as they get closer to death. We just need to speed that process along. Sort of what I am hoping your ex-husband will help us do."

Ellen, now surprised, said, "Vinnie. What does Vinnie have to do with your warped ideas?"

"Well, Ellen, what I know about human nature is that rich or poor, smart or uneducated, anyone will do anything for love or money if they are desperate enough. Vinnie, I think, is desperate enough to do anything to save his brother-in-law and maybe, in his booze-soaked mind, win you back."

Remembering a text message she received the other day from a friend at the club about seeing Vinnie and Alex in a heated argument, Ellen pressed Alex further, "What did you do with Vinnie? Tell me, Alex."

"That information, my dear Ellen, will require you to do something for me."

"Like what?" Ellen said warily.

"I need you to collaborate my story that it was Kenny who ordered the killings of those people, not me. If you do, it will be our word against Kenny and the gang bangers. Hell, I even had those thugs use Kenny's car with my spare key when he was at the Cardinals games, so it would look like he was involved in every one of these crimes. No one will believe him and the gang bangers. Secondly, you will back me with the investors and the board. Knowing you and I are in lockstep on this will give them the backbone to put their muscle to thwart any investigations or pin the murders on Kenny and the gang bangers. The board will need to make a nice million-dollar donation to the police union and some politicians to make it all go away, but that is a small price for their payoff in a few years."

Without sounding too eager, Ellen said, "And if I do this, if I back you, you will get Vinnie out of whatever trouble he may be in?"

"Yes," Alex said. "Plus, if we are in lockstep, I will double your shares, assuming I remain CEO."

"And you will promise me that no loose ends tie you to any of these murders?" Ellen asked.

"No more loose ends. I have taken care of everyone," Alex said, his eyes black, in contrast to the subtle undetectable smile on his face knowing that Ellen and Vinnie were new loose ends he would be dealing with soon.

Ellen left knowing a secret, as well. She would not bend to Alex's ridiculous plan and was recorded on the wire she was wearing not under her blouse but as one of her earrings. However, she needed to find Vinnie quickly to make sure whatever idea Alex put in Vinnie's head would end now.

CHAPTER 67

Listening to the conversation between the wired-up Dr. Calabrese and Alex Finnegan, Rhonda knew she had ample evidence to arrest Alex Finnegan in his office immediately after Ellen left. However, since he was a very connected guy, she went to a judge to get a search warrant for Alex Finnegan's home, car, and office, including his cellphone and computer. With the warrant in hand, she would head down to arrest Alex Finnegan, and this time, regardless of how many people he would try to pay off, she hoped he would be convicted of these crimes.

But Rhonda had a more immediate concern after hearing the vague information about Ellen's ex-husband Vinnie. She needed to track him down and understand what he may be up to. It was a small world that Dr. Calabrese's ex-husband was the witness to the hit and run of Brian Coffman in Forest Park. Rhonda had suspicions about Vinnie back then, and this new information troubled her. She did not have time to chase down Vinnie, so she went to the second floor of the precinct to meet with Ally Moloney, the street cop working on the Brian Coffman case.

"Hey, Moloney. Remember about eight weeks ago when you and I were on the scene for the hit and run in Forest Park, a young guy named Brian Coffman, hit while riding his bike?"

"Sure, Detective, what's up?" Moloney responded eagerly.

"Well, the guy we interviewed at the scene that we thought was kind of odd, I need you to follow up with him on something."

Going through her computer screens to get back to that case, Moloney found the witness's name and read it out loud, "Vinnie Calabrese, witness, drove black Honda truck. Lives on Edwards Street."

Rhonda nodded and told Moloney, "We need to track him down quickly. I have to arrest a suspect in the murder case I am working on. So, grab your partner, run down to Mr. Calabrese's home, and see if he is there. If he is there, do not engage. Just call me back and let me know what you find."

Ally turned off her computer and signaled to her partner to meet her out at the car.

CHAPTER 68

It had been two days since Vinnie hit Jonas Stecker with his truck, and it seemed for nothing as Frank was still in the hospital waiting for a match. Stecker either was still alive or died without using his organs. Frank had been in the hospital for about five days, and Vinnie remembered Frank's transplant coordinator, Brooke MacIntosh, telling him most patients, once they are in the hospital sick enough to get a transplant, need to get one in 10-12 days. *How many days did Frank have?* Vinnie wondered. He knew it wasn't long, but Vinnie only had one more name on his list that could save Frank. In his deteriorating mindset, Vinnie still believed he was doing the right thing, thinking: *if I go down, I am going down fighting for Frank.* Looking for updated news on Stecker, he went to type Stecker's name into the Post-Dispatch search bar but stopped when he saw this headline and story:

Black Honda Pickup Truck Sought in Soulard Hit and Run.

Clicking on the story, Vinnie read,

"Police are asking people to report any information they may have on a late model black Honda Ridgeline pickup truck that may be involved in a hit and run of Mr. Jonas Stecker near 9th and Sidney Street at approximately 11:30 p.m., in the Soulard area. Information can be reported at 1-866-371-8477 (TIPS). Mr. Stecker remains in critical but improving condition at Barnes-Jewish hospital.

Vinnie stared at his phone, stunned. It was only a matter of time before the cops tracked him down, not only for the truck's description but now the poor decision to make what he thought was an anonymous 911 call reporting the hit and run on Stecker. He assumed the police could trace the call back to his phone and then to him. He knew he did not have much time before being picked up. Looking at his watch, he saw it was around 10:00 a.m., and he remembered that Marvin Applebaum went to the Botanical Garden every Wednesday at 10:00. What he planned to do was risky, but he had no choice. He was in this all the way, and however it ended, it ended. Vinnie took out his gun from his dresser drawer, packed it in his pants, and then headed off to the Botanical Gardens, which was only a few blocks from his home. As he jumped in the driver's seat, he did not notice the scrapes on the passenger side front bumper that showed silver flakes from Jonas Stecker's bike frame. He also certainly did not see the blood splatters from Stecker that blended into Vinnie's black truck.

CHAPTER 69

Vinnie parked on Magnolia Avenue, a street bordering the southern part of the park near the employee entrance of the Botanical Gardens. He wanted an escape route as what he needed to do would be more difficult if he had to take Marvin Applebaum out of the main gate past the security guards. As Vinnie entered the park, he walked along all the paths looking for a large group of elderly people on a tour. He knew Marvin and his fellow residents would probably have a guide or aides with them. After about 15 minutes of walking, he came upon a large group of slowly moving elderly men and women, and in the group, he spotted Marvin. He needed to isolate him and do it in an area that was as close as possible to the employee exit where Vinnie parked his car. The group entered the Japanese Garden, a beautiful part of the park and a favorite of many visitors with its manicured stone gardens, bonsai trees, and Koi ponds where young and old would buy pellets to feed the very large and always ravenous Koi.

This area would be the perfect place to whisk Marvin away as everyone's attention would be looking over the bridge into the water as the fish swam to the top, jostling each other as their large mouths inhaled the food pellets tossed to them.

Just like managing a group of children, the aides were busy with their elderly charges, buying the pellets from the dispenser, ensuring each resident had a handful, and asking people to move aside so all the elderly residents could get a better feeding spot.

As Marvin drifted a few feet away from the group, Vinnie grabbed Marvin's arm and began slowly steering him down the path away from the Koi area. He seemed to recognize Vinnie's face from his visit to the assisted living center, but to make sure, Vinnie reminded him of that visit.

"Marvin, so nice to see you. It's me, Tom Riley. Remember we talked at your apartment?"

"Oh, yes, Tom. So nice to see you. Is your brother here with you?"

"He is Marvin. I told him you would be here, and he told me he would love to see you and give you a private behind-the-scenes tour of the English Woodland Garden. They have some fabulous new plantings, and he would love to show them to you."

"Oh, that would be wonderful. You know I am originally from England and how I miss the English Gardens." He walked blissfully with Vinnie, farther and farther away from the group until they got to a side path deeper into the woods and out of sight from the group. He just needed to walk him out of the back gate before anyone noticed he was missing. Coming up to the maintenance building in the back of the park, Vinnie slipped through the gate and onto Magnolia Avenue, undetected by any of the staff and seemingly oblivious to Marvin, who had severe enough dementia and was easily led astray. Vinnie came up to his truck and said, "Marvin, it's easier to drive to the main entrance. It'll be a lot less walking for you, so let me get you settled in, and I will have you in the beautiful English countryside in a few minutes." Marvin got in. Vinnie buckled his seatbelt. Ironic, he thought, because he would not need it in about 10 minutes, and they headed off to Forest Park. Vinnie needed Marvin as close as possible to the Barnes trauma center and Frank.

As they pulled away, Vinnie did not notice a gardener on lunch break following them as they went beyond the employee exit. He found it very odd that two visitors would try to exit the Garden from the back rather than the main entrance. It seemed to him that the younger man, while not overly aggressive, was very paranoid, looking around as he guided the older man to his car. The gardener had an elderly father himself, and when he was with him, he had to pay attention to his every footstep so he would not fall. But as he watched, it seemed Vinnie was more concerned about his surroundings than the sure footing of his companion. He was unsure why it all seemed suspicious, but he decided to take a photo of Vinnie's truck and license plate and report what he saw to the Garden's security team.

CHAPTER 70

Police officer Ally Moloney got to Vinnie's house on the Hill and saw no sign of his pick-up truck and no sign of Vinnie. The house seemed locked up and unoccupied. She called Detective Simon to tell her the status and await Rhonda's instructions. As she waited in her car, she heard over her scanner an announcement of a possible abduction from The Missouri Botanical Gardens of an elderly man, white, bald, in his late 60s to early 70s. The man was taken out of a rear entrance by a man they believed to be Vincent Calabrese, owner of a black Honda pickup truck with Missouri license plate UB4MAN. As she debated her next move, Rhonda called her back.

"Ally," Rhonda said urgently, "there is an ABP out on Vinnie Calabrese. He has abducted a man named Marvin Applebaum, and we believe he plans to harm him. I have a call into his ex-wife to see if she has heard from Vinnie or if she may be able to track his whereabouts based on his phone location. Just stay at his house in case he comes back there."

Rhonda had a shitload of problems to deal with. When she went to arrest Alex Finnegan at his office, she was told by his assistant that he had an unexpected business trip to the United Arab Emirates and he would be out of the office for the next two weeks. Rhonda knew the UAE did not have an extradition treaty with the United States, and she knew it would be difficult to get Finnegan arrested and sent back.

Rhonda's pursuit with Finnegan had only just begun, and her guess is it would soon involve the FBI and our embassy in the UAE. Rhonda guessed Finnegan took a boat load of investor money and had set up his backup plan and possibly another transplant operation in the UAE. She also thought that as shrewd as Finnegan was, he probably had his escape route planned long in advance as the UAE was a wealthy enclave with the end-of-life and transplant viewpoints aligned with Finnegan. Guys like Finnegan always had a backup plan and always seemed to stay away from the U.S. court system.

Locally though, she had other problems because, at the end of the day, Rhonda was a St. Louis cop trying to prevent the murders of St. Louis citizens. The citizens she was most concerned about at this very moment were Vinnie Calabrese and Marvin Applebaum. With a sense of extreme urgency, Rhonda tracked down Dr. Calabrese to give her an update on Vinnie and his actions at the Botanical Garden.

"Dr. Calabrese, do you have any idea where Vinnie may be taking this man?" Rhonda asked.

"I think I do. It is the one place where he would go to think things out, usually while fishing or walking. Forest Park. Most likely Jefferson Lake. Ever since we divorced, he would go there, sometimes to fish or think, but I know it was to gaze up to my apartment building. He told me once that it was the one way he still felt connected to me. That is where I would go, Detective. Please find him before he hurts that poor man or even himself."

CHAPTER 71

Vinnie walked around Jefferson Lake with Marvin, his gun hidden in his waistband. If all went well, the small 22-caliber bullet would not kill Marvin instantly but do enough damage to put him on life support, and in less than 24 hours, due to his dementia and age, he would likely be giving his organs to those in need, especially Frank. Marvin was such a kind old man. He had no idea where he was and no idea he was minutes away from death. All he kept talking about was seeing the old English gardens he loved so much. As they walked around the trails of Jefferson Lake, Vinnie kept up the charade, telling Marvin that these were the English Gardens. Disoriented, he cheerfully went along.

They walked around the lake, where Vinnie had spent so much time fishing and people-watching. He always marveled at the quietness of the lake, contrasting with the traffic noises and the sounds of ambulances and medivac helicopters making hourly runs to Barnes hospital only 200 yards in the distance. Vinnie was always at peace in the park and at the lake, yet he would wonder about the hell people in that hospital, including Frank, were going through. They were suffering death and sickness while he was free to live a healthy life. It just did not seem fair to Vinnie for him to have his life and others, like Frank, maybe to lose theirs. But Marvin Applebaum would change all that. Dementia had taken the last years of his life. Marvin had lived a good one, Vinnie assumed. Now he would be making the last great gift of his life. But Vinnie needed to make sure Marvin's body would be found quickly to get him to Barnes and prepare for the transplant for Frank.

Assuming it would take paramedics about 5 minutes to get to him, Vinnie called 911, said his location, and then hung up. A minute later, he heard the sirens, hoping as soon as they arrived to discover Marvin's body, Frank would be on his way to getting his lungs. Vinnie looked in the direction of Barnes Hospital, where Frank lay fighting for his life, and Vinnie, in his mind, thought he was going to finally do something great with his life. Vinnie raised the gun behind Marvin's head and then turned to look at the police rushing towards him. He pulled the trigger.

Detective Simon and the other police moved in on Vinnie, guns drawn, yelling for him to put the gun down. The quietness of the park was broken by the sounds of gunshots, which echoed from the park to the hospital complex and back. Once the echo ended, the sound that took over was that of the police and EMT converging on Vinnie and Marvin. Vinnie had finally done something great with his life, something he had wanted to do all along. Save Frank.

CHAPTER 72

The Christmas season was very special to Frank and Sue, especially this year, as Frank was recovering nicely from his lung transplant several months ago. All his children and grandchildren were with him as they celebrated the annual Christmas Eve dinner of Seven Fishes and plates of Italian delicacies. This year the gathering was larger than most as Frank invited members of his transplant team to enjoy Sue's cooking as he constantly talked about it to them. Many stopped by, including Brooke MacIntosh, who felt honored to be invited as she had become very close with the Esposito family and had taken a liking to Benjamin, one of Frank and Sue's sons. He also invited Vinnie's children, his three nieces, and his ex-wife, Ellen, to come as they had had a very tough time lately because of Vinnie's death. Ellen could not make it because she was giving a speech in Washington about breakthroughs the Arch City Transplant Center had made in transplant success. As their new CEO, she was on Capitol Hill trying to drum up support for new legislation in the transplant business. As Frank led the assembled in prayer before eating, he thought about and prayed for Vinnie. He thought about how much he missed him and the violent tragedy that had ended his life. Frank thought he would surely be the one dying, not Vinnie, but God always has his own plans.

As grace ended and everyone settled down for the delicious feast, the doorbell rang. Frank went to answer the front door. As he opened it, Frank was greeted by their mail carrier, Larry Gaylord, who had a registered letter from the National Transplant Organization. Frank figured it was the usual survey or solicitation for money that he got constantly.

Wishing Larry a Merry Christmas, Frank opened the envelope and read the letter, but he stopped, stunned, five lines in.

Dear Mr. Esposito,

> *As you requested to know who your donor was, the deceased's family has given the National Transplant Organization permission to release your donor's name. Upon your authorization, we will provide the donor family with your name and facilitate a meeting if you and the donor family desire to meet. Your donor who was a perfect match for you was:*
>
> *Mr. Vincent Calabrese, Age upon death: 64*
>
> *Cause of Death: Blunt Head Trauma caused by gunshot*
>
> *We hope you stay in good health, Mr. Esposito. If you choose to contact the donor's family, please respect their loss and understand that while a life was gained, a life was lost.*

Sincerely,
Roy Carroll
President of The National Transplant Organization

Frank put the letter in his pocket and returned to his family and their other guests, including Vinnie's children, all enjoying their Christmas Eve dinner. Before serving the food, Frank offered a toast to Vinnie, staring intently into the eyes of Vinnie's children as he gave it, wondering if they knew what a hero their father was. As Frank enjoyed the Angels Wings more than any other Christmas, he would think of Vinnie, knowing how much Vinnie would have enjoyed them as well.

The End

PERSONAL REFLECTION FROM FRANK ZUCCARELLI, THE REAL-LIFE FRANK ESPOSITO FROM "THE PERFECT MATCH."

I was diagnosed with Interstitial Lung Disease in October of 2018. This disease reduces your quality of life, and as it progresses, it reduces it even more. I was not a smoker, nor did I work in any environmentally hazardous areas. The official diagnosis came from the doctors at Barnes Jewish Hospital in St. Louis, Missouri. At first, I was shocked that my situation was this serious, but I felt I needed to do what was necessary to be approved for a lung transplant. The results of extensive testing qualified me for a transplant with the caveat of losing weight. I was then placed on the waiting list.

I would like to express my deepest appreciation for the brilliant lung transplant teams at Barnes Jewish Hospital. The many pre-transplant, transplant, and post-transplant doctors, nurses, therapists, and staff were crucial in my care, healing, and recovery. Their skills, knowledge, encouragement, and compassion were instrumental in supporting me through the entire lung transplant process.

The disease progressed rapidly throughout that year. Every month I needed to increase my oxygen needs to maintain the appropriate oxygen saturation level. I struggled physically with basic everyday tasks like walking, taking showers, and sleeping. I could no longer participate in activities with my family, grandchildren, or friends. Throughout this, I do not remember being scared or afraid of dying. My only goal was to make it through each day and then the next, taking the necessary steps to be ready for the transplant. I had faith that God was providing me guidance and a path, regardless of the direction it would take me.

I had wonderful support from my primary caregiver, an angel of a wife, my children and daughter-in-law, Vinnie Calabrese and Dr. Ellen-James Calabrese (aka Steve and Nancy Pizzolato), and the rest of my family and friends. As my primary caregiver, my wife, Sue, went above and beyond to help me cope, heal, and be encouraged throughout the various stages of my disease, and her devotion and love were, and are, something I will be thankful for forever. I had my transplant on May 15th, 2019, after the doctors found my "Perfect Match." At this point, I want to express my deepest gratitude to the donor family for their generosity and all donor families who have also shared a part of their loved ones to save the life of another. My donor was a 31-year-old woman in prison. Her family has given me a second chance at life, for without her lungs, I would not be living the life I am today. As this book accurately portrays my challenges and significant health decline with this disease, I cannot stress enough the importance of being an organ donor and how organ donation can improve and impact the lives of others more than you can imagine.

I take care of my new lungs by eating right, exercising regularly, practicing martial arts, and often wearing a mask. Organ rejection is one of the potential eventual outcomes that an organ recipient can be diagnosed with which could reduce the organ's viability and/or recipient's life span. Ongoing research on organ rejection will improve the longevity of organ recipients. The proceeds of this book will be supporting that effort.

I thank God, my donor family, the Barnes Jewish Hospital team, and the many prayers every day for a second chance. God blessed me with a new life, no longer needing oxygen, enjoying simple things like playing with my grandchildren, going to dinner with family and friends, and even doing household chores. Every day is a blessing. Cherishing the activities I do with my family and friends is a joy. I appreciate life itself more than ever. A second chance has given me more patience, understanding, and compassion for others. I try not to be bothered by the trivial issues that come my way. This journey has given me a new perspective on situations and a greater love for life. I appreciate every day I have with the people I love, and I will forever be thankful for my "Perfect Match."

Letter to Donor Family from Frank Zuccarelli

Dear Donor Family,

My name is Frank, and I received the lungs from your family member. I would like to express my deepest sympathies for your loss. I have lost several family members, and I understand how difficult this time can be. I am a religious person, so I believe they are in a better place with God. I still think of my parents, who have been deceased for over 20 years, but I believe they are happier in heaven with God. I also find comfort in the good memories I have shared with my parents. I hope you can do the same with your loved one.

I cannot express my gratitude for the decision you made to donate your loved one's lungs. You have given me another chance in life. I had a form of Interstitial Lung Disease called IPF, Idiopathic Pulmonary Fibrosis. It is a lung disease that scars your lungs. As the disease progresses, it becomes more difficult to breathe. I had the disease for about a year. I was required to take oxygen tanks everywhere I went. As the year progressed, I needed more and more oxygen. Then ten days before my transplant on May 15th, I was admitted to the hospital because I could not provide myself with enough oxygen at home. It has been a challenging journey. God and prayers have helped me throughout this journey. I am currently in a rehabilitation program to increase my lung capacity and strengthen my body. It is going well.

I am a 60-year-old man with a wife, three children, and two grand-children. Your gift has allowed me to enjoy my family again. I now appreciate every moment I spend with them even more than before. I have learned to re-prioritize what is important in life. I can now do things with them. God and my family are the most important things in my life. I can continue to work and provide for my family. I love to go to plays, concerts, and dinner with my family. I have three older boys who I can still teach about life. My oldest has grandchildren, who we help babysit. My middle son wants to start a business, so I can help him with that. My youngest son is in college. This week we are going to look for apartments. I can enjoy and swim in our pool. I can teach my grandchildren how to swim. My 3-year-old grand-daughter is in dance recitals that I can now go to. I have a 6-month-old grandson that I can hold and feed. These are all precious moments that I treasure, thanks to you.

I pray and think of your family and your loss. Every day I thank God for the decision you made to give me another chance at life. It is the greatest gift one could give to another person. God bless you and your family. You will always be in my prayers.

Pre-transplant
Before the Double Lung Transplant Surgery

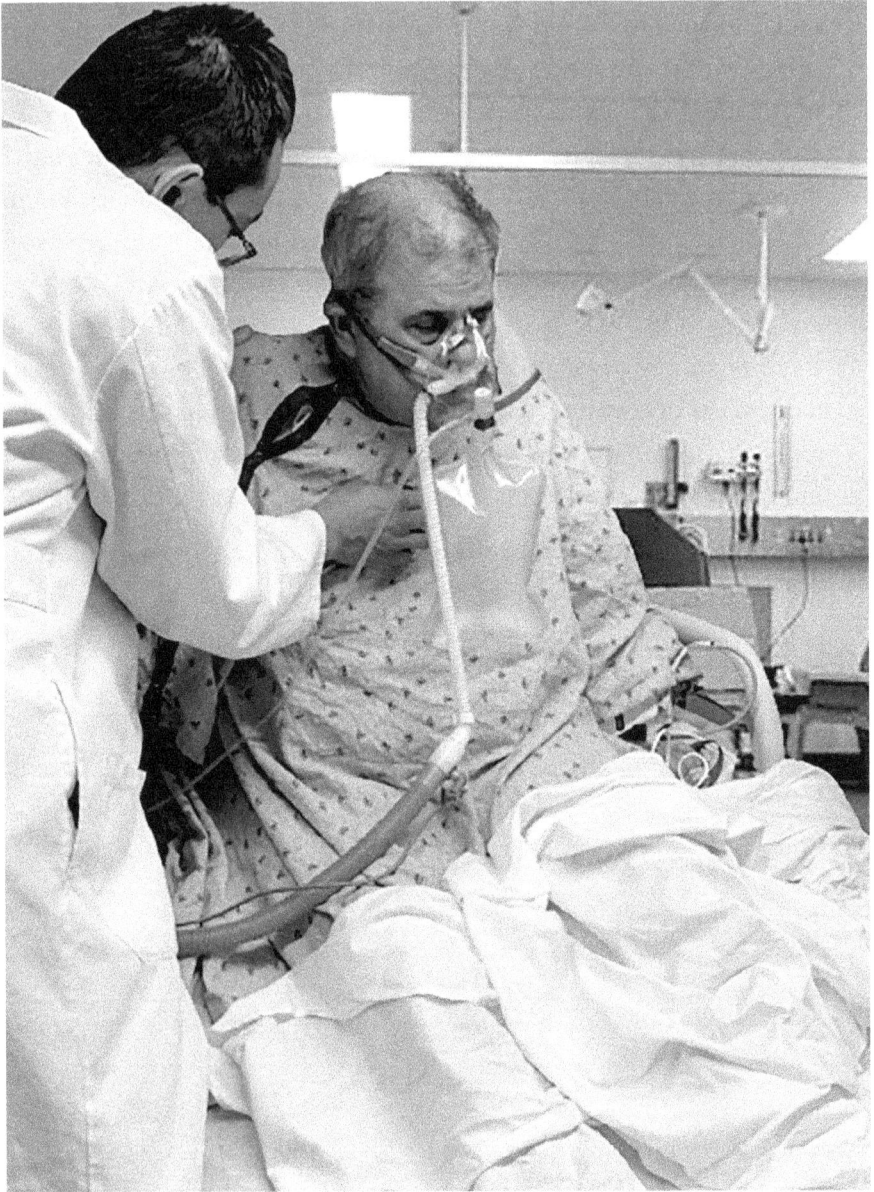

60th Birthday Party

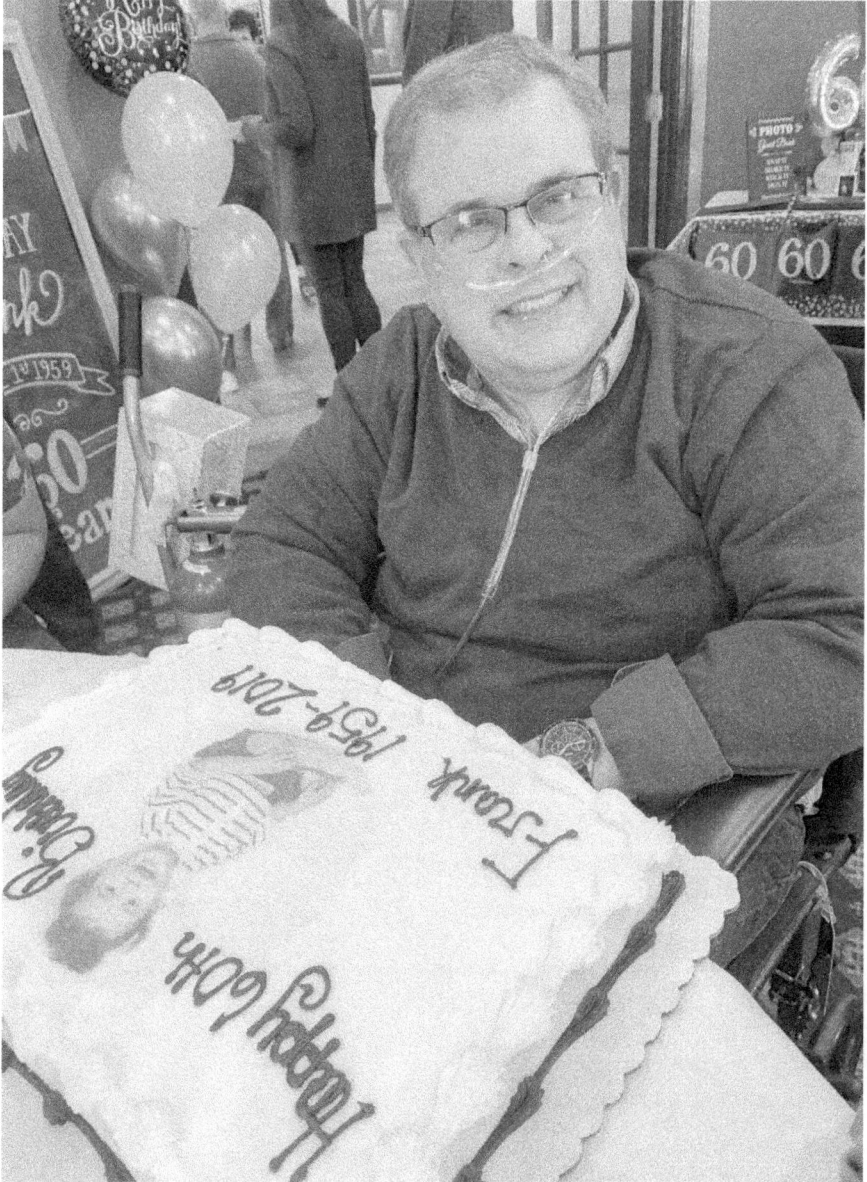

Post-transplant

In Recovery and Intubated Post Double Lung Transplant Surgery

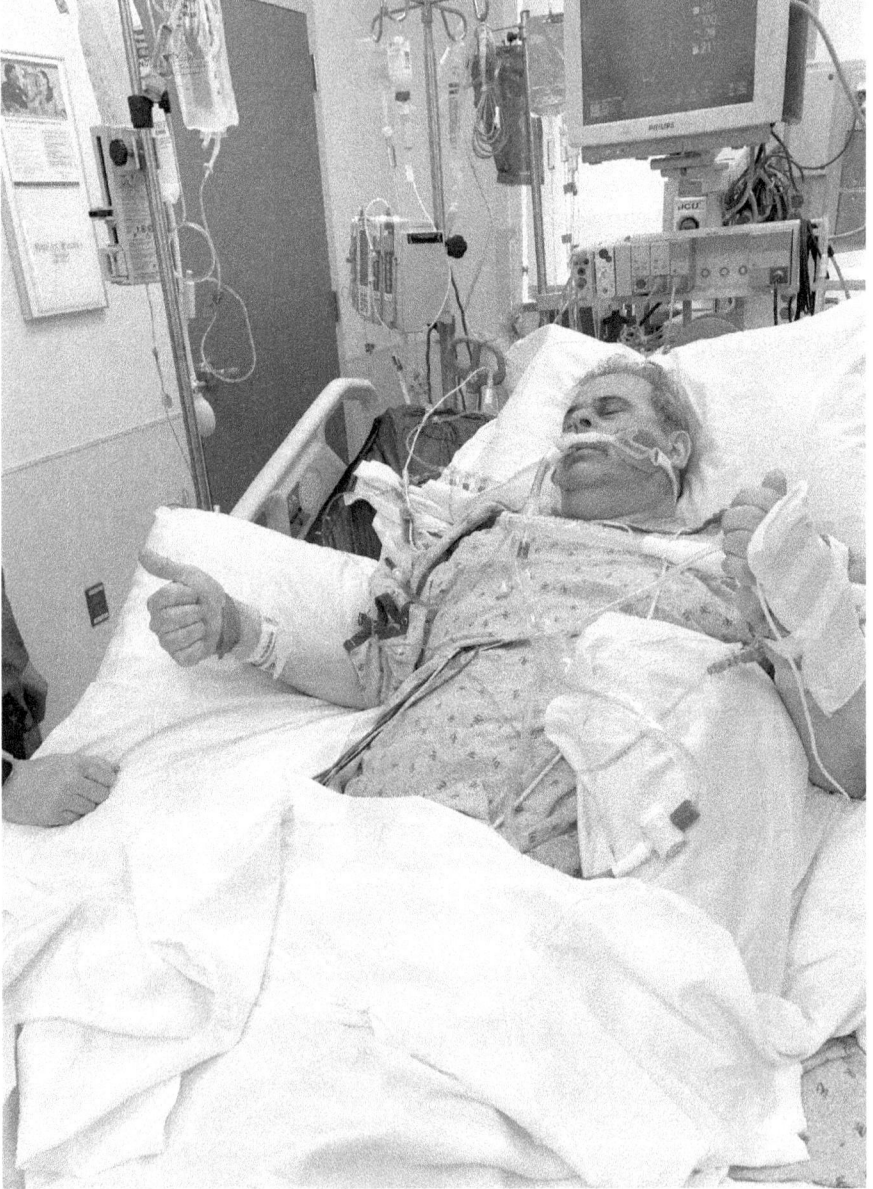

Steve Pizzolato

In Recovery

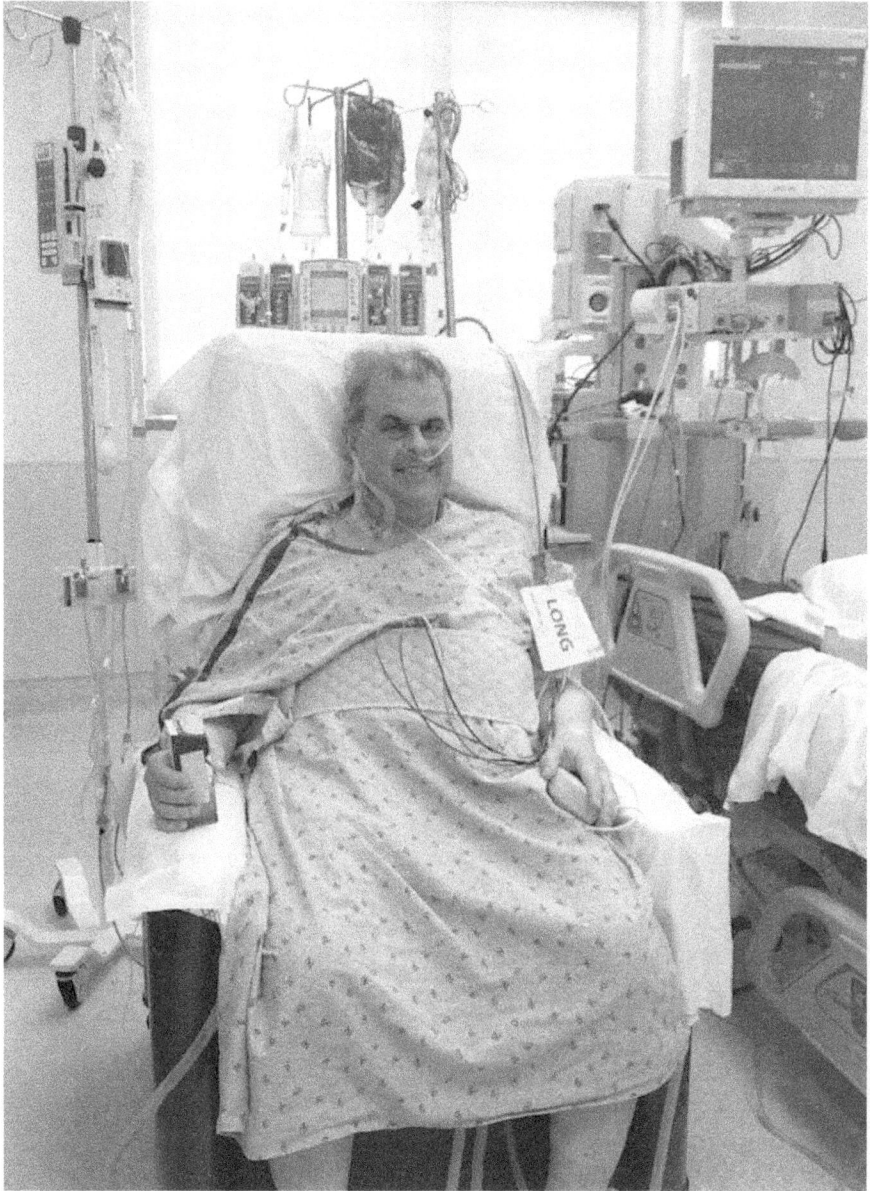

Frank and Sue, on The Hill, St. Louis Three Months Post Transplant

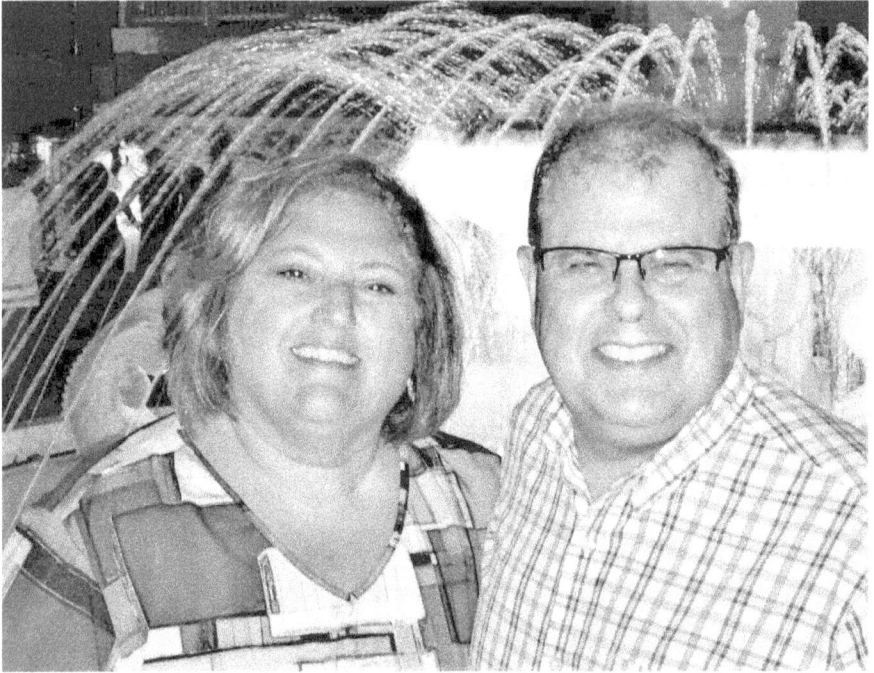

Three Months Post Transplant with
Nancy, Steve, Sue, and Frank on The Hill, St. Louis

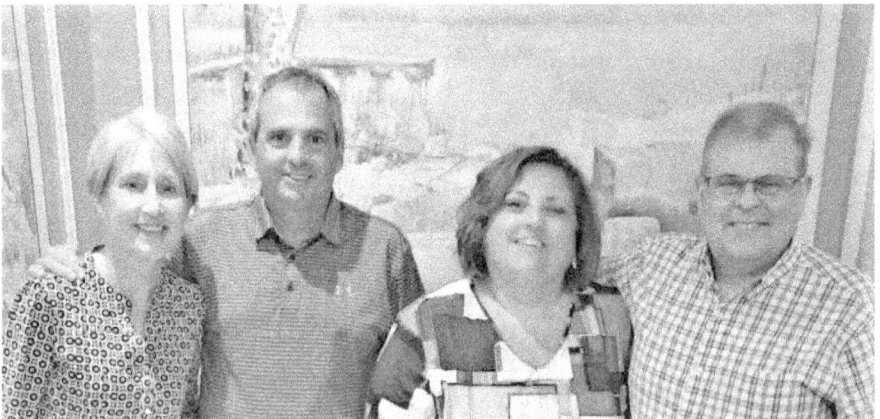

Steve Pizzolato

One Year Double Lung Transplant Anniversary

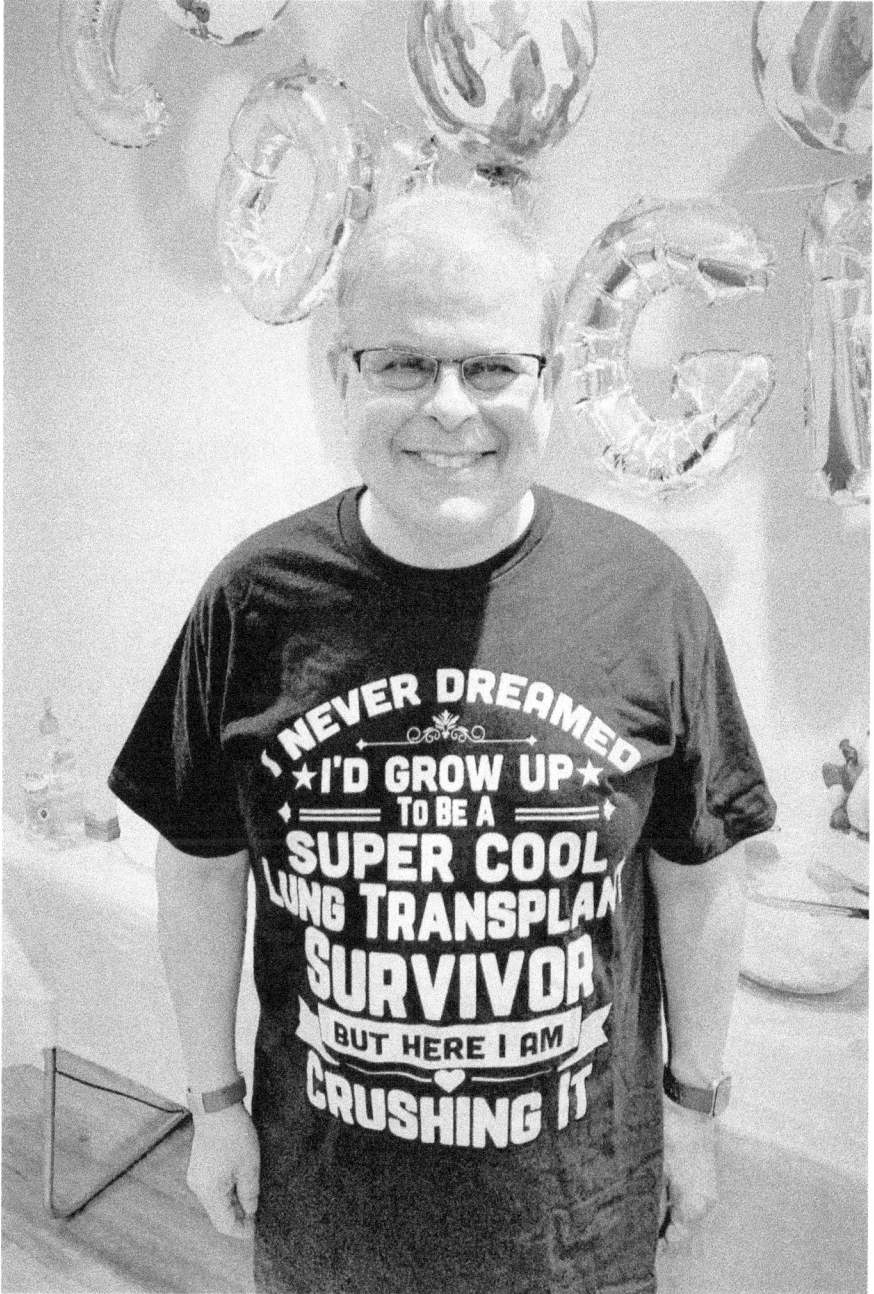

50% of the profits of *The Perfect Match* will be donated to Barnes-Jewish Hospital for the lifesaving work they do every day and to the United Network for Organ Sharing (UNOS), which performs a valuable service of finding and matching donors to those in need of a transplant.

If you enjoyed *The Perfect Match* and want to donate to Barnes-Jewish Hospital, please go to: https://www.foundationbarnesjewish.org/How-to-Give. If you want to learn more about or donate to UNOS, please visit https://unos.org/.

NOAH'S ARK
PREVIEW OF THE NEXT BOOK IN
THE PERFECT MATCH SERIES

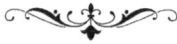

CHAPTER 1

"**N**oah, get off your ass and clean up the damn monkey cages. Then feed them!" Noah's supervisor at the St. Louis Zoo yelled at him.

"Jesus, Lou, get off my back. I'll do it in a minute," Noah angrily replied.

He wanted to finish reading and comment on an article he had just read on his phone. Noah's fans demanded to hear his opinion, and no matter what an asshole Lou was, Noah had to take the time to provide a thoughtful response to his fans. They expected it from Noah. Once done with his response, Noah got up, grabbed a shovel and a broom, and headed towards the primate cages. As he walked to the cages, Noah thought to himself how much more he liked the primates than he did his co-workers, especially Lou, his overbearing boss of the last five years.

While Noah had no close relationships with people, he had a special bond with the monkeys he kept fed and whose cages he kept clean. Noah understood animals, especially monkeys. Eat, Sleep, Shit, Sex. That was a monkey's life. In a way, he was jealous of the simplicity in their lives. They even looked forward to seeing people, especially Noah, as his arrival for first cleaning the cage, followed by feeding the monkeys, was a daily ritual both man and beast looked forward to. Noah had worked at the zoo for nearly 20 years since graduating from community college with an associate degree in exotic animal training and management. His plan was to go on to fulfill his desire to get a zoology degree at the University of Missouri. But that plan fizzled out as most of Noah's plans did, despite being labeled as a genius with a reported 150 IQ. At 41, Noah, genius or not, had reached the pinnacle of his career – if cleaning monkey shit could be called a career. But Noah never cared about his career trajectory as he set his bar low in his teenage years, and it had not been raised or exceeded. His personal life was no better than his career. He had no one in his life. No wife, no girlfriend, no family. Noah had come to grips that this was his life. Lonely.

But that was fine for Noah, as he, in his mind, had an online family. He was a significant influencer in people's everyday lives as Noah primarily spent most of his time posting comments on sports stories. Still, occasionally he would comment on local or world events. The commentary handle he used at the St. Louis Post-Dispatch was NoahItAll. A clever play on words, he thought, on his full name, Noah Sharpe, and his belief that he did know it all. His fellow commenters thought he was clever as many of them liked or highlighted his comments, which Noah thought made him quite an important online influencer. Noah believed he had true fans as people seemed to listen to what he had to say about sports and life. He primarily commented on the pitching and hitting woes of the Cardinals, the goal-scoring woes of the Blues, or the lack of offense or defense for the area's college teams. In Noah's mind, he should be on a sports radio station or TV as a sportscaster, but Noah knew those jobs went to ex-athletes, women, or mandatory minority hires. Noah was better than all of them, he thought, and whenever he went to sports memorabilia shows where athletes or the media would gather, he would always try to engage in conversations with them, trying to impress them with his vast knowledge of sports. However, they usually pulled away from the conversation sooner than Noah would have liked. *"Pompous assholes,"* Noah thought as they hurried away from him. Everyone it seemed in Noah's life sped away or ghosted him. He silently accepted it and his fate, but he hoped for something more in his mind.

CHAPTER 2

❦

Dr. Layla Brazini was always the first to work at the New Beginnings Fertility Clinic. And being first to work meant being at work at 5:00 am as she wanted to get in her workout at the facility's private fitness center she installed when she started the clinic 15 years ago. As soon as she arrived, she noticed something amiss as the door to her private entrance to the clinic, while closed now, had been obviously tampered with earlier as she could see what looked like crowbar marks embedded between the door and the doorframe.

"Dammit, she thought, had I not set the alarm before I left last night?"

She proceeded with some trepidation, unsure if the intruders were waiting for her in her office or clinic. She opened the door and turned on the lights, but not before she released the safety on her gun that she always kept in her purse. While Dr. Brazini's life's work helped facilitate life for those who could not conceive, she was savvy enough to understand a gun may be the only way to protect her life in the job and city she was in. Years ago, a doctor was respected and usually untouchable by crime, much like a policeman, teacher, or social worker. Not anymore, unfortunately.

As she walked into her office, she immediately saw what little files she had on her desk, strewn on the floor. No patient information was ever kept in a hard copy file, so she ignored the mess and looked down at her desk, noticing that the drawers the desk contained were busted wide open. Again, knowing nothing significant was ever kept in those drawers, she was not too concerned about what might have been taken, maybe some tickets to a theater event or petty cash. The thieves would be disappointed if this was a robbery for personal items or items that could be hocked for money or drugs. Leaving her office, she went into the medical areas of the clinic, and what she saw alarmed her greatly and indicated the thieves were both sophisticated and focused on the most valuable items in the clinic. The frozen embryos!

While the freezer doors were busted open, the area holding the embryos was not trashed as she thought it would be or as a vandal might do, but it seemed to her that each embryo chamber was carefully removed with almost no damage. Removed as cleanly as one of her lab technicians would do.

"But why and who," she wondered.

From time to time, she knew the clinic was a target of religious zealots and protesters who thought conception should not be done scientifically. They were still against the use of IVF despite it being salvation for nearly 50 years for women who could not conceive naturally. Most of the time, the protesters stayed on the street and left in peace after a few hours of yelling. But she also knew that with Roe vs. Wade, a topic as heated as it has ever been, being challenged nationally and by the states, IVF clinics, and the embryos, more specifically, the discarding of unused embryos, were being questioned. She had received communications from ASRM, The Association of Reproductive Medicine, that IVF clinics may be targeted by protesters and future regulations.

Something beyond her logical comprehension had happened at her clinic. She needed to report it to the police immediately, but she did not want them storming in and treating it as a routine robbery. She wanted to first consult with someone she trusted who knew would look beyond the obvious. She picked up her phone and dialed perhaps the one cop she did trust or least used to during the most critical years of her life. Detective Rhonda Simon.

CHAPTER 3

Her three-month suspension ended as the investigators had determined that St. Louis Detective Rhonda Simon had correctly acted in her handling of the attempted murder of Marvin Applebaum by Vinnie Calabrese. Never mind that Simon probably saved Applebaum's life; the fact that she killed the suspect before he could kill himself or Applebaum caused the protesters and the media to demand an investigation and the immediate suspension of Simon, a 30-year veteran on the force. Simon felt she should not have been suspended. But she was being served up as an example of how the police and the government officials would have a zero-tolerance policy for cops involved in questionable shootings.

The time of the suspension, though, was a godsend for Simon. She was burnt out. 2021 was brutal in St. Louis with murders and crime. Although the final numbers were on track to be slightly below 2020. In addition to her daily caseload witnessing and solving the depravity and viciousness of ordinary St. Louis citizens, the big case she had in her grasp soon eluded her, partly because of the suspension but mainly because of the suspect. Dr. Alex Finnegan had fled the country and landed in the UAE.

The case, featuring multiple murders covering up past crimes and newer murders to aid in an organ donation scheme, had become the responsibility of the FBI and the SEC. Dr. Finnegan had also absconded with millions of dollars of investor money intended to grow Finnegan's vision of the Arch City Transplant Center.

Simon was hours away from putting the cuffs on Finnegan for a crime that now had made national and international news. A crime so big that Simon might have ridden it, and the notoriety to become police commissioner or mayor of St. Louis. But Finnegan was gone, leaving Simon as only a footnote and foot soldier to a bigger story.

However, Rhonda Simon did not wallow in self-pity for the three months she was suspended, as she spent most of that time in the powerful arms and soft bed of Richard Leary, the former private investigator. His research had helped Simon solve the Finnegan case. Most cops who are suspended and under investigation hit the bottle. And Simon, in her past, had done her share of drinking. So alcohol did not interest her as a stress reliever. Sex, lots of it, did the trick for Simon.

Richard Leary fit the bill for now, but Rhonda Simon had no interest in anything more than a few laughs and a lot of sweaty nights. Maybe Leary thought more of their relationship, but they had not reached the point of having that uncomfortable conversation discussing where the relationship was headed. Regardless of the state of her personal life, Simon was excited to restart her professional life and hit the streets of St. Louis, where rampant crime would provide her with another kind of stimulation.

But this morning, hitting the sheets with Richard one more time became more enticing than hitting the streets and catching bad guys. However, as she was about to be taken by Richard, her phone buzzed, and she knew from the name listed only as "HER," identifying the caller, this was the only person who might be able to get her out of bed and out of Richard Leary's arms. She paused for a moment, thinking perhaps about the last time "HER" had passed in and out of Rhonda's life, and with both trepidation and a bit of nostalgic tingling inside, answered, "Layla. It's been too long."

CHAPTER 4

At 36, Becca Stevens felt she was running out of time. But Becca Stevens never would run out of options. She was determined to achieve her goals, and no door would ever be closed to her. Becca had given up on getting married. She was not a lesbian, but at this point in her life, she hated men. Especially men who seemed entitled to tell her what she could and could not do with her mind or body. But unfortunately, to have a baby, she needed a man, or at least a by-product of the only thing a man was good for, in her mind, his sperm for procreation. She had decided to start a family by going to an IVF clinic and having her eggs implanted with anonymous sperm from a sperm donor bank. While researching the processes, philosophy, success rates, and costs of IVF centers around the United States, Becca chose New Beginnings Fertility Clinic in her hometown, St. Louis. New Beginnings was not the least expensive. In fact, with an upfront fee of $40,000, it was on the upper end of costs for comparable options. Money was not a concern to Becca as she was a successful entrepreneur who had started a women's swimwear line several years ago, now generating 15 million dollars in revenue. She had also turned down several offers three times that amount because she still loved the business and really had no other interests in life beyond that. But having a baby would change all that, and Becca thought that if her IVF treatments were successful, perhaps having a baby would change her priorities on what she wanted to spend her time on.

So, after doing all her research on IVF centers, the deciding factors for Becca were two things. One, New Beginnings, specialized in single women or gay women who wanted to start a family but needed a sperm donor. And two, the dynamic and almost hypnotic personality of the owner of New Beginnings, Dr. Layla Brazini, who Becca had met at a Women in Leadership conference six months previously. While in different businesses and slightly different age groups, Layla Brazini was 40 and Becca 36, they clicked immediately upon meeting. It seemed they had the same drive regarding business and the emerging role of women as business leaders. They also were aligned culturally and politically. They both believed in women having more choice in their own lives, including income equality, if not superiority, if they outworked men, which they regularly did. They also had little use for men in their lives. Though Layla was completely open regarding her sexual preferences, Becca was just at a point where men she had dated had failed to reach the intelligence, maturity, and open-mindedness Becca was looking for in a partner.

Becca knew she was making a life-changing decision going through IVF, and she knew the only person she could trust to guide her through the process was Dr. Layla Brazini, whose New Beginning Center now possessed Becca's most precious gift, her unfertilized eggs. They would stay frozen at New Beginnings until Becca chose the best sperm for fertilization.

About the Author

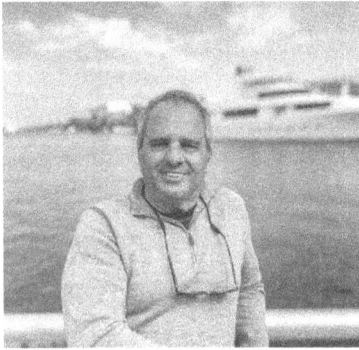

Steve Pizzolato is originally from Chicago but has lived in St. Louis for most of his life. Steve comes from a large Italian American family with seven brothers and sisters and over 30 nieces and nephews. He met and married his wife, Nancy, of 40 years, in St. Louis. Together, they have three daughters and three grandsons. Steve acquired his love of reading and writing from his mother, who was a librarian. Before publishing *The Perfect Match*, Steve owned a successful digital marketing agency for 21 years. He's an avid and talented fisherman, an enthusiastic but mediocre golfer, and a passionate foodie, especially regarding the delicious food at the many Italian restaurants St. Louis has to offer.

www.ingramcontent.com/pod-product-compliance
Lightning Source LLC
Chambersburg PA
CBHW021849020426
42334CB00013B/254